Anti-Inflammatory Diet Meal Prep Cookbook

The Beginner's Guide to Clean and Delicious Prep-and-Go Recipes to Reduce Inflammation, Optimize Gut Health, and Heal the Immune System

Amanda K. Sanders

Table of Contents

Chapter 1: An Introduction to Anti-Inflammatory Eating

Understanding Inflammation

Inflammation is a natural and essential process in the body. It serves as a defense mechanism, safeguarding our bodies from infections, injuries, and toxins. When the body detects harmful stimuli, it initiates an inflammatory response, mobilizing white blood cells to the affected areas and facilitating healing. This inflammation is vital for our health.

However, issues arise when inflammation becomes long-lasting or chronic. In contrast to acute inflammation, which is temporary and subsides once the threat is eliminated, chronic inflammation persists over time. Several factors can contribute to this, such as an unhealthy diet, high levels of stress, lack of physical activity, and exposure to harmful environmental substances. Chronic inflammation has been associated with several health problems, including heart disease, diabetes, arthritis, and certain types of cancer.

Understanding the difference between acute and chronic inflammation is crucial for recognizing the significance of managing inflammation through lifestyle choices, especially diet. By embracing an anti-inflammatory diet, we can support our bodies in fighting chronic inflammation and reducing the risk of associated health conditions.

The Benefits of Following an Anti-Inflammatory Diet

An anti-inflammatory diet aims to include foods that can effectively reduce and prevent chronic inflammation. This way of eating can result in a wide range of health benefits, including:

1. Reduced Risk of Chronic Diseases: An anti-inflammatory diet is high in nutrients that decrease the risk of chronic diseases like heart disease, diabetes, and certain cancers. Certain foods, such as leafy greens, berries, and fatty fish, have compounds that can effectively reduce inflammation within cells.

2. Improved Digestive Health: Prolonged inflammation has the potential to harm the gut lining, resulting in digestive problems such as irritable bowel syndrome (IBS) and leaky gut syndrome. An anti-inflammatory diet supports gut health by including fiber-rich foods and probiotics, which help maintain a healthy microbiome.

3. Improved Immune Function: An anti-inflammatory diet can strengthen the immune system by reducing chronic inflammation. This enhanced immune function can improve the body's ability to combat infections and illnesses.

4. Improved Weight Management: Chronic inflammation is frequently linked to increased body weight and obesity. An anti-inflammatory diet, which emphasizes whole, nutrient-dense foods, can help with weight loss and maintenance by improving metabolic function and reducing inflammation-related weight gain.

5. Improved Mental Health: There is a correlation between inflammation and mental health conditions like depression and anxiety. Foods with anti-inflammatory properties, particularly those high in omega-3 fatty acids, antioxidants, and vitamins, can improve brain health and mood.

6. Healthy Aging: Chronic inflammation speeds up aging and plays a role in age-related diseases. A diet that reduces inflammation can support the health of the body's cells and tissues, contributing to a longer and more vibrant life.

Essential Anti-Inflammatory Foods

Incorporating anti-inflammatory foods into your diet is a highly effective way to address chronic inflammation. Here are some of the most beneficial foods to include:

1. Leafy Greens: Vegetables like spinach, kale, and Swiss chard are rich in antioxidants and vital nutrients that help reduce inflammation. In addition, they contain a significant amount of fiber, which is beneficial for maintaining a healthy gut.

2. Berries: Various berries, such as blueberries, strawberries, raspberries, and blackberries, contain antioxidants, specifically anthocyanins, which possess potent anti-inflammatory properties.

3. Fatty Fish: Salmon, mackerel, sardines, and trout are excellent choices for obtaining omega-3 fatty acids, linked to reducing inflammation and promoting heart health.

4. Nuts and Seeds: Almonds, walnuts, chia seeds, and flaxseeds are packed with healthy fats, fiber, and antioxidants that help fight inflammation.

5. Olive Oil: Extra virgin olive oil is commonly included in anti-inflammatory diets because of its rich concentration of monounsaturated fats and polyphenols, known for their potent anti-inflammatory properties.

6. Turmeric: This spice is known for its vibrant yellow color and contains curcumin, a compound with strong anti-inflammatory and antioxidant properties. Including turmeric in your meals can significantly reduce inflammation.

7. Ginger: Ginger is well-known for its anti-inflammatory and antioxidant properties, which can help reduce inflammation and pain. It is widely used in cooking and beverages.

8. Green Tea: Packed with polyphenols and antioxidants, green tea has been proven to have anti-inflammatory properties and offer a wide range of health benefits.

9. Garlic: Garlic contains sulfur compounds that have anti-inflammatory properties. It also boosts the immune system and helps fight infections.

10. Tomatoes: Tomatoes are rich in vitamin C, potassium, and lycopene, an antioxidant known for its anti-inflammatory properties, mainly when cooked.

11. Whole Grains: Foods like quinoa, brown rice, and oats are rich in fiber and essential nutrients that promote a healthy gut and lower inflammation.

By incorporating these anti-inflammatory foods into your meal prep routine, you can make tasty and nourishing meals that promote your overall health and well-being. The upcoming chapters will offer practical advice and recipes to assist you in starting your anti-inflammatory journey.

Chapter 2: Meal Prep Fundamentals

Getting Started with Meal Prep

Meal prepping is an organized method of planning and preparing your meals ahead of time. It saves time and guarantees that you will have healthy, anti-inflammatory meals ready for the entire week. Here's a step-by-step guide to help you begin:

1. Plan Your Meals: Start deciding on the meals you want to prepare for the week. It is crucial to include a range of anti-inflammatory foods in your diet while maintaining a balanced intake of proteins, healthy fats, and carbohydrates. Design a comprehensive menu featuring breakfast, lunch, dinner, and snack options.

2. Make a Shopping List: After finalizing your menu, create a comprehensive shopping list that includes all the necessary ingredients. Arrange your list according to different grocery store sections (such as produce, pantry, dairy, etc.) to enhance the efficiency of your shopping trip.

3. Schedule Prep Time: Set aside a designated time for meal prepping, such as a weekend morning or evening. Allocate 2-3 hours of your time to prepare and cook your meals for the entire week effectively. Establishing a regular meal prep routine can make it a habit.

4. Start Simple: If you're new to meal prepping, start with simple recipes that require minimal ingredients and preparation. As you gain confidence, you can gradually incorporate more complex meals and diversify your menu.

5. Batch Cooking: Prepare generous amounts of staple foods such as grains, proteins, and vegetables that you can use in multiple recipes. For instance, prepare a large quantity of quinoa or brown rice, roast a tray of mixed vegetables, and grill several chicken breasts. These ingredients can be combined in various ways to make multiple meals throughout the week.

6. Portion Control: Use portion control containers to separate your meals into individual servings. This not only makes it convenient to grab a meal on the go but also helps manage portion sizes and prevent overeating.

Essential Kitchen Tools and Equipment

Having the proper tools and equipment significantly improves the efficiency of meal prepping. Here are a few essential items to consider:

1. Quality Knives: A reliable collection of sharp knives is essential for effectively chopping, slicing, and dicing. This includes a chef's knife, paring knife, and serrated knife.

2. Cutting Boards: Use separate cutting boards for vegetables, meats, and bread to prevent any potential cross-contamination. Choose boards that are durable and easy to clean.

3. Mixing Bowls: Various-sized mixing bowls can be handy for combining ingredients, marinating meats, and making salads.

4. Measuring Cups and Spoons: Precise measurements are crucial for recipes, particularly when baking. Consider purchasing a set of measuring cups and spoons.

5. Food Processor and Blender: These appliances are efficient for chopping, pureeing, and blending, making meal preparation quicker and easier. They are handy for making smoothies, sauces, and dips.

6. Sheet Pans and Baking Dishes: High-quality sheet pans and baking dishes are essential for tasks such as roasting vegetables, baking proteins, and preparing casseroles.

7. Nonstick Skillets and Pots: Consider investing in nonstick skillets and pots. They can make cooking a variety of dishes easier and require less oil.

8. Storage Containers: For storing prepped meals, it is important to have storage containers that are BPA-free and microwave-safe. Find a wide range of sizes and shapes to suit various types of food.

9. Instant Pot or Slow Cooker: These appliances effortlessly prepare generous portions of food. They are excellent for soups, stews, and other one-pot meals.

10. Spice Rack: A properly stocked spice rack allows you to add flavor and anti-inflammatory benefits to your meals without the need for excessive salt or harmful additives.

Storage Tips and Techniques

Ensuring proper storage is crucial for maintaining the freshness and safety of your prepped meals. Here are some helpful tips and techniques to keep your meals tasting delicious all week long:

1. Cool Before Storing: Allow hot foods to cool to room temperature before transferring them to storage containers. This helps to prevent condensation, which can result in food becoming soggy and promote the growth of bacteria.

2. Use Airtight Containers: Store your meals in airtight containers to ensure their freshness and prevent unwanted odors from permeating the refrigerator. Glass containers are an excellent choice because of their durability and odor resistance.

3. Label and Date: Remember to label your containers with the contents and the date they were prepared. This will help you stay organized and keep track of when you made the dish. This process allows you to easily monitor the duration of food storage, ensuring that you enjoy your meals when they are at their freshest.

4. Refrigerate or Freeze: Store prepped meals in the refrigerator if you plan to consume them within 3-4 days. To ensure meals stay fresh for extended periods, store them in freezer-safe containers. Remember to leave some room at the top of the container because liquids tend to expand when they freeze.

5. Reheat Safely: Reheat your meals thoroughly to eliminate any possible bacteria by ensuring they reach an internal temperature of 165°F (74°C). Reheat only the portion you plan to eat to maintain the quality of the remaining food.

6. Rotate Your Meals: Follow the "first in, first out" approach, consuming older meals before newer ones. This helps minimize waste and ensures that you can enjoy your meals at their freshest.

Chapter 3: 30-Day Meal Plan

Day	Breakfast	Lunch	Dinner	Snack
1	Quinoa and Sweet Potato Breakfast Casserole	Lemon-Herb Grilled Turkey Breast	Chili-Lime Tofu and Broccoli Stir-Fry	Pomegranate and Pistachio Quinoa Salad
2	Mixed Berry and Almond Overnight Oats	Grilled Vegetable and Quinoa Stuffed Portobello Mushrooms	Herb-Crusted Mahi-Mahi with Roasted Vegetables	Avocado and Tomato Cucumber Rolls
3	Zucchini and Spinach Egg Muffins	Pesto-Marinated Grilled Shrimp Skewers	Sweet Potato and Chickpea Coconut Curry	Berry Avocado Salsa with Cinnamon Tortilla Chips
4	Chia Seed Pudding Parfait with Berries	Spinach and Feta Stuffed Quinoa Peppers	Baked Turmeric Chicken Thighs with Brussels Sprouts	Turmeric-Carrot Muffins with Coconut Glaze
5	Mixed Berry and Spinach Smoothie Bowl	Avocado and Black Bean Lettuce Wraps	Turmeric-Cashew Chicken Skewers	Golden Milk Chia Pudding Parfait
6	Turmeric-Coconut Milk Smoothie Bowl	Walnut-Crusted Chicken Tenders with Zucchini Noodles	Harissa-Marinated Lamb Kebabs with Quinoa Tabouleh	Berry Chia Seed Jam
7	Turmeric-Spiced Sweet Potato Soup	Tomato and Basil Quinoa Risotto	Greek Yogurt Marinated Chicken Kabobs with Tzatziki	Cucumber and Avocado Gazpacho
8	Turmeric and Cumin Roasted Carrots	Sesame-Crusted Ahi Tuna with Spinach Salad	Grilled Turmeric Tofu Skewers	Roasted Red Pepper and Lentil Patties
9	Mixed Berry and Quinoa Breakfast Casserole	Blackened Tilapia with Mango-Avocado Salsa	Quinoa and Chickpea Curry	Mango-Turmeric Lassi with Mint
10	Berry and Walnut Quinoa Salad	Green Tea Poached Chicken with Bok Choy	Spaghetti Squash Primavera with Basil Pesto	Almond-Crusted Halibut with Mango Salsa
11	Golden Turmeric Cauliflower Rice	Teriyaki Salmon and Quinoa Lettuce Wraps	Roasted Garlic and Herb Quinoa Patties	Berry and Coconut Yogurt Parfait
12	Blackberry and Mint Infused Water	Avocado and Chickpea Stuffed Bell Peppers	Walnut-Crusted Chicken Salad with Raspberry Vinaigrette	Lemon-Garlic Roasted Broccoli and Cauliflower

13	Turmeric and Cinnamon Baked Apples	Cilantro-Lime Chicken and Avocado Salad	Oven-Roasted Cod with Tomato-Olive Relish	Brussels Sprouts and Almond Stir-Fry
14	Coconut-Curry Almond Butter Stir-Fry	Miso-Glazed Sea Bass with Sesame Green Beans	Tandoori-Style Chicken Skewers with Cucumber Raita	Lemon-Garlic Roasted Broccoli and Cauliflower
15	Berry and Almond Butter Smoothie	Quinoa and Edamame Salad with Miso Dressing	Pistachio-Crusted Cod with Lemon-Dill Aioli	Coconut Turmeric Shrimp Stir-Fry
16	Strawberry and Avocado Quinoa Bowl	Roasted Beet and Goat Cheese Salad	Roasted Red Pepper and Quinoa Stuffed Zucchini Boats	Turmeric-Lime Coconut Energy Bites
17	Raspberry and Almond Baked Salmon	Ginger-Soy Glazed Salmon with Asparagus	Coconut-Curry Cashew Chicken	Artichoke and Spinach Stuffed Mushrooms
18	Caprese Avocado Toast with Balsamic Glaze	Grilled Chicken Salad with Berry Vinaigrette	Turmeric-Spiced Quinoa Patties	Roasted Turmeric Cauliflower Steaks
19	Mixed Berry Sorbet with Mint	Avocado and Blueberry Spinach Salad with Hemp Seeds	Lemon-Herb Grilled Turkey Breast	Roasted Garlic and Herb Quinoa Patties
20	Blueberry and Kale Salad with Lemon Poppyseed Dressing	Ginger-Turmeric Quinoa Stir-Fry	Herb-Crusted Mahi-Mahi with Roasted Vegetables	Turmeric and Coriander Roasted Chickpeas
21	Mixed Berry and Almond Overnight Oats	Spicy Ginger-Orange Glazed Tempeh	Cilantro-Lime Chicken and Avocado Salad	Walnut and Cranberry Stuffed Acorn Squash
22	Avocado and Tomato Cucumber Rolls	Cumin-Spiced Quinoa and Black Bean Bowl	Rosemary-Dijon Baked Pork Chops with Cauliflower Mash	Berry Chia Seed Jam
23	Berry and Walnut Stuffed Acorn Squash	Walnut-Crusted Chicken Tenders with Zucchini Noodles	Turmeric-Cashew Chicken Skewers	Lemon-Garlic Roasted Broccoli and Cauliflower
24	Mixed Berry and Spinach Smoothie Bowl	Pesto-Marinated Grilled Shrimp Skewers	Sweet Potato and Chickpea Coconut Curry	Berry Avocado Salsa with Cinnamon Tortilla Chips
25	Golden Turmeric Cauliflower Rice	Sesame-Crusted Ahi Tuna with Spinach Salad	Turmeric-Spiced Sweet Potato Soup	Roasted Red Pepper and Lentil Patties
26	Quinoa and Sweet Potato Breakfast Casserole	Lemon-Herb Grilled Turkey Breast	Green Tea Poached Chicken with Bok Choy	Pomegranate and Pistachio Quinoa Salad

27	Zucchini and Spinach Egg Muffins	Walnut-Crusted Chicken Salad with Raspberry Vinaigrette	Chili-Lime Tofu and Broccoli Stir-Fry	Berry Chia Seed Jam
28	Mixed Berry and Almond Overnight Oats	Grilled Vegetable and Quinoa Stuffed Portobello Mushrooms	Herb-Crusted Mahi-Mahi with Roasted Vegetables	Avocado and Tomato Cucumber Rolls
29	Chia Seed Pudding Parfait with Berries	Spinach and Feta Stuffed Quinoa Peppers	Baked Turmeric Chicken Thighs with Brussels Sprouts	Turmeric-Carrot Muffins with Coconut Glaze
30	Mixed Berry and Spinach Smoothie Bowl	Avocado and Black Bean Lettuce Wraps	Turmeric-Cashew Chicken Skewers	Golden Milk Chia Pudding Parfait

Chapter 4: Quinoa Recipes

Quinoa and Roasted Vegetable Buddha Bowl

Prep Time: 20 minutes | **Cook Time:** 30 minutes | **Servings:** 4

Ingredients:

- 1 cup quinoa, rinsed
- 2 cups broccoli florets
- 1 large sweet potato, peeled and cubed
- 1 red bell pepper, sliced
- 1 yellow bell pepper, sliced
- 1 medium zucchini, sliced
- 1 tablespoon olive oil
- 1 teaspoon ground turmeric
- 1 teaspoon ground cumin
- 1 teaspoon paprika
- 1/2 teaspoon garlic powder
- 1/2 teaspoon onion powder
- Salt and pepper to taste
- 2 cups baby spinach
- 1 avocado, sliced

Instructions:

1. Preheat the oven to 400°F (200°C).

2. In a large bowl, combine broccoli, sweet potato, red bell pepper, yellow bell pepper, and zucchini. Drizzle with olive oil and toss to coat. Add turmeric, cumin, paprika, garlic powder, onion powder, salt, and pepper. Toss again to evenly coat the vegetables.

3. Spread the seasoned vegetables in a single layer on a baking sheet. Roast in the preheated oven for 25-30 minutes or until the vegetables are tender and slightly crispy at the edges.

4. While the vegetables are roasting, rinse quinoa under cold water. Cook quinoa according to package instructions.

5. Once the quinoa and vegetables are ready, assemble the Buddha bowls. Divide cooked quinoa among four bowls. Top each with a portion of roasted vegetables, a handful of baby spinach, and sliced avocado.

6. Serve immediately, or store in airtight containers for a heart-healthy, low-sodium, and anti-inflammatory meal prep option.

Nutritional Information (per serving):

- Carbs: 45g
- Sodium: 150mg
- Fats: 15g
- Protein: 10g

Mediterranean Quinoa Salad with Lemon-Tahini Dressing

Prep Time: 15 minutes | **Cook Time:** 15 minutes | **Servings:** 4

Ingredients:

- 1 cup quinoa, rinsed
- 2 cups cherry tomatoes, halved
- 1 cucumber, diced
- 1/2 cup Kalamata olives, pitted and sliced
- 1/2 cup red onion, finely chopped
- 1/2 cup fresh parsley, chopped
- 1/4 cup fresh mint, chopped
- 1/3 cup feta cheese, crumbled
- 1/4 cup extra-virgin olive oil
- 3 tablespoons tahini
- 3 tablespoons fresh lemon juice
- 1 clove garlic, minced
- Salt and pepper to taste

Instructions:

1. Rinse quinoa under cold water. In a medium saucepan, combine quinoa with 2 cups of water. Bring to a boil, then reduce heat to low, cover, and simmer for 15 minutes or until quinoa is cooked and water is absorbed. Fluff with a fork and let it cool.

2. In a large bowl, combine cooled quinoa, cherry tomatoes, cucumber, Kalamata olives, red onion, parsley, mint, and feta cheese.

3. In a small bowl, whisk together olive oil, tahini, lemon juice, minced garlic, salt, and pepper to create the dressing.

4. Pour the lemon-tahini dressing over the quinoa mixture. Toss gently to ensure all ingredients are evenly coated.

5. Divide the salad into four meal prep containers. Store in the refrigerator for a heart-healthy, low-sodium, and anti-inflammatory meal prep option.

Nutritional Information (per serving):

- Carbs: 40g
- Sodium: 200mg
- Fats: 15g
- Protein: 10g

<u>Spinach and Feta Stuffed Quinoa Peppers</u>

Prep Time: 20 minutes | **Cook Time:** 30 minutes | **Servings:** 4

Ingredients:

- 4 large bell peppers, halved and seeds removed
- 1 cup quinoa, rinsed
- 2 cups fresh spinach, chopped
- 1/2 cup red onion, finely chopped
- 1 clove garlic, minced
- 1 tablespoon olive oil
- 1 teaspoon dried oregano
- 1 teaspoon dried basil
- Salt and pepper to taste
- 1 cup feta cheese, crumbled
- 1 can (14 ounces) diced tomatoes, drained

Instructions:

1. Preheat the oven to 375°F (190°C).

2. In a medium saucepan, combine quinoa with 2 cups of water. Bring to a boil, then reduce heat to low, cover, and simmer for 15 minutes or until quinoa is cooked and water is absorbed. Fluff with a fork and let it cool.

3. While quinoa is cooking, heat olive oil in a pan over medium heat. Add chopped spinach, red onion, and minced garlic. Sauté until the spinach is wilted and the onions are translucent. Add dried oregano, dried basil, salt, and pepper. Stir to combine.

4. In a large bowl, mix cooked quinoa, sautéed spinach mixture, crumbled feta cheese, and drained diced tomatoes.

5. Place bell pepper halves in a baking dish. Stuff each pepper half with the quinoa mixture.

6. Cover the baking dish with foil and bake in the preheated oven for 25-30 minutes, or until the peppers are tender.

7. Let the stuffed peppers cool before transferring them to meal prep containers for storage. Store in the refrigerator for a heart-healthy, low-sodium, and anti-inflammatory meal prep option.

Nutritional Information (per serving):

- Carbs: 35g
- Sodium: 250mg
- Fats: 15g
- Protein: 10g

Citrusy Quinoa Pilaf with Almonds

Prep Time: 15 minutes | **Cook Time:** 20 minutes | **Servings:** 4

Ingredients:

- 1 cup quinoa, rinsed
- 2 cups low-sodium vegetable broth
- 1 orange, zest, and juice
- 1 lemon, zest, and juice
- 1 tablespoon olive oil
- 1/2 cup red onion, finely chopped
- 1/2 cup carrot, diced
- 1/4 cup almonds, sliced
- 1 teaspoon ground turmeric
- 1 teaspoon ground cumin
- Salt and pepper to taste
- 1/4 cup fresh cilantro, chopped
- 1/4 cup dried cranberries

Instructions:

1. In a medium saucepan, combine quinoa and low-sodium vegetable broth. Bring to a boil, then reduce heat to low, cover, and simmer for 15 minutes or until quinoa is cooked and liquid is absorbed. Fluff with a fork and let it cool.

2. In a large skillet, heat olive oil over medium heat. Add chopped red onion, diced carrot, and sliced almonds. Sauté until the vegetables are tender and the almonds are lightly toasted.

3. Add ground turmeric, ground cumin, salt, and pepper to the skillet. Stir to coat the vegetables and almonds with the spices.

4. In a small bowl, whisk together the zest and juice of the orange and lemon.

5. Add the cooked quinoa to the skillet, pouring the citrus mixture over it. Stir until well combined and heated through.

6. Remove the skillet from heat and fold in chopped fresh cilantro and dried cranberries.

7. Allow the citrusy quinoa pilaf to cool before transferring it to meal prep containers. Store in the refrigerator for a heart-healthy, low-sodium, and anti-inflammatory meal prep option.

Nutritional Information (per serving):

- Carbs: 40g
- Sodium: 200mg
- Fats: 10g
- Protein: 8g

Roasted Red Pepper and Quinoa Stuffed Zucchini Boats

Prep Time: 20 minutes | **Cook Time:** 25 minutes | **Servings:** 4

Ingredients:

- 2 large zucchini
- 1 cup quinoa, rinsed
- 2 cups low-sodium vegetable broth
- 1 cup roasted red peppers, diced
- 1/2 cup red onion, finely chopped
- 2 cloves garlic, minced
- 1 tablespoon olive oil
- 1 teaspoon dried oregano
- 1 teaspoon dried basil
- Salt and pepper to taste
- 1/2 cup feta cheese, crumbled
- 1/4 cup fresh parsley, chopped

Instructions:

1. Preheat the oven to 375°F (190°C).
2. Cut the zucchini in half lengthwise. Scoop out the seeds, creating a hollow space for the stuffing.
3. Place the zucchini halves on a baking sheet, cut side up.
4. In a medium saucepan, combine quinoa and low-sodium vegetable broth. Bring to a boil, then reduce heat to low, cover, and simmer for 15 minutes or until quinoa is cooked and liquid is absorbed. Fluff with a fork and let it cool.
5. In a skillet, heat olive oil over medium heat. Add chopped red onion and minced garlic. Sauté until the onions are translucent.
6. Add diced roasted red peppers, dried oregano, dried basil, salt, and pepper to the skillet. Stir to combine.
7. Combine the cooked quinoa with the red pepper mixture. Fill each zucchini boat with the quinoa and red pepper stuffing.
8. Top each stuffed zucchini boat with crumbled feta cheese.
9. Bake in the preheated oven for 20-25 minutes, or until the zucchini is tender.
10. Garnish with fresh parsley before serving. Allow the stuffed zucchini boats to cool before storing them in meal prep containers. Store in the refrigerator for a heart-healthy, low-sodium, and anti-inflammatory meal prep option.

Nutritional Information (per serving):

- Carbs: 35g
- Sodium: 180mg
- Fats: 10g
- Protein: 8g

<u>Ginger-Turmeric Quinoa Stir-Fry</u>

Prep Time: 15 minutes | **Cook Time:** 20 minutes | **Servings:** 4

Ingredients:

- 1 cup quinoa, rinsed
- 2 cups low-sodium vegetable broth
- 2 tablespoons olive oil
- 1 tablespoon fresh ginger, minced
- 2 cloves garlic, minced
- 1 cup broccoli florets
- 1 cup carrot, julienned
- 1 red bell pepper, sliced
- 1 yellow bell pepper, sliced
- 1 zucchini, sliced
- 1 teaspoon ground turmeric
- 1 teaspoon ground coriander
- 1 teaspoon soy sauce (low-sodium)
- Salt and pepper to taste
- 1/4 cup fresh cilantro, chopped
- 1/4 cup unsalted cashews, chopped

Instructions:

1. In a medium saucepan, combine quinoa and low-sodium vegetable broth. Bring to a boil, then reduce heat to low, cover, and simmer for 15 minutes or until quinoa is cooked and liquid is absorbed. Fluff with a fork and let it cool.

2. In a large skillet or wok, heat olive oil over medium-high heat. Add minced ginger and garlic, sautéing until fragrant.

3. Add broccoli florets, julienned carrots, sliced red and yellow bell peppers, and sliced zucchini to the skillet. Stir-fry until the vegetables are crisp-tender.

4. Sprinkle ground turmeric, ground coriander, low-sodium soy sauce, salt, and pepper over the vegetables. Toss to coat evenly.

5. Add the cooked quinoa to the skillet. Stir-fry for an additional 3-4 minutes until the quinoa is well combined with the vegetables.

6. Remove the stir-fry from heat and fold in chopped fresh cilantro.

7. Allow the ginger-turmeric quinoa stir-fry to cool before transferring it to meal prep containers. Top each serving with chopped unsalted cashews.

8. Store in the refrigerator for a heart-healthy, low-sodium, and anti-inflammatory meal prep option.

Nutritional Information (per serving):

- Carbs: 40g
- Sodium: 150mg
- Fats: 10g
- Protein: 8g

Quinoa and Kale Patties with Avocado Sauce

Prep Time: 20 minutes | **Cook Time:** 25 minutes | **Servings:** 4

Ingredients:

For the Patties:

- 1 cup quinoa, rinsed
- 2 cups low-sodium vegetable broth
- 2 cups kale, finely chopped
- 1/2 cup red onion, finely chopped
- 2 cloves garlic, minced

- 1 teaspoon ground cumin
- 1 teaspoon ground coriander
- Salt and pepper to taste
- 2 eggs, beaten
- 1/4 cup whole wheat flour

For the Avocado Sauce:

- 1 ripe avocado, peeled and pitted
- 1/4 cup Greek yogurt

- 1 tablespoon fresh lemon juice
- 1 tablespoon fresh cilantro, chopped
- Salt and pepper to taste

Instructions:

1. In a medium saucepan, combine quinoa and low-sodium vegetable broth. Bring to a boil, then reduce heat to low, cover, and simmer for 15 minutes or until quinoa is cooked and liquid is absorbed. Fluff with a fork and let it cool.

2. In a large bowl, combine cooked quinoa, finely chopped kale, finely chopped red onion, minced garlic, ground cumin, ground coriander, salt, and pepper.

3. Add beaten eggs and whole wheat flour to the quinoa mixture. Mix well until all ingredients are evenly combined.

4. Shape the mixture into patties, using about 1/4 cup for each.

5. Heat olive oil in a skillet over medium heat. Cook the quinoa and kale patties for 3-4 minutes on each side, or until golden brown and cooked through.

6. For the avocado sauce, combine ripe avocado, Greek yogurt, fresh lemon juice, chopped fresh cilantro, salt, and pepper in a blender. Blend until smooth.

7. Serve the quinoa and kale patties with a dollop of avocado sauce.

8. Allow the patties to cool before transferring them to meal prep containers. Store in the refrigerator for a heart-healthy, low-sodium, and anti-inflammatory meal prep option.

Nutritional Information (per serving):

- Carbs: 35g
- Sodium: 180mg

- Fats: 15g
- Protein: 10g

<u>Pomegranate and Pistachio Quinoa Salad</u>

Prep Time: 15 minutes | **Cook Time:** 15 minutes | **Servings:** 4

Ingredients:

- 1 cup quinoa, rinsed
- 2 cups low-sodium vegetable broth
- 1 cup pomegranate arils
- 1/2 cup pistachios, shelled and chopped
- 1 cucumber, diced
- 1/4 cup red onion, finely chopped
- 1/4 cup fresh mint, chopped
- 1/4 cup feta cheese, crumbled
- 2 tablespoons extra-virgin olive oil
- 1 tablespoon balsamic vinegar
- Salt and pepper to taste

Instructions:

1. In a medium saucepan, combine quinoa and low-sodium vegetable broth. Bring to a boil, then reduce heat to low, cover, and simmer for 15 minutes or until quinoa is cooked and liquid is absorbed. Fluff with a fork and let it cool.

2. In a large bowl, combine cooked quinoa, pomegranate arils, chopped pistachios, diced cucumber, finely chopped red onion, chopped fresh mint, and crumbled feta cheese.

3. In a small bowl, whisk together extra-virgin olive oil, balsamic vinegar, salt, and pepper.

4. Pour the dressing over the quinoa mixture and toss to combine, ensuring even coating.

5. Allow the salad to chill in the refrigerator for at least 30 minutes to let the flavors meld.

6. Before serving, toss the salad once more and adjust salt and pepper to taste.

7. Portion the salad into meal prep containers for a heart-healthy, low-sodium, and anti-inflammatory meal prep option.

Nutritional Information (per serving):

- Carbs: 35g
- Sodium: 180mg
- Fats: 15g
- Protein: 8g

Quinoa and Sweet Potato Breakfast Casserole

Prep Time: 20 minutes | **Cook Time:** 40 minutes | **Servings:** 6

Ingredients:

- 1 cup quinoa, rinsed
- 2 cups low-sodium vegetable broth
- 2 medium sweet potatoes, peeled and diced
- 1 tablespoon olive oil
- 1 onion, finely chopped
- 2 cloves garlic, minced
- 1 red bell pepper, diced
- 1 green bell pepper, diced
- 1 teaspoon ground turmeric
- 1 teaspoon smoked paprika
- Salt and pepper to taste
- 6 large eggs
- 1 cup unsweetened almond milk
- 1/2 cup feta cheese, crumbled
- Fresh parsley, chopped (for garnish)

Instructions:

1. In a medium saucepan, combine quinoa and low-sodium vegetable broth. Bring to a boil, then reduce heat to low, cover, and simmer for 15 minutes or until quinoa is cooked and liquid is absorbed. Fluff with a fork and let it cool.

2. Preheat the oven to 375°F (190°C).

3. In a large skillet, heat olive oil over medium heat. Add finely chopped onion and minced garlic. Sauté until the onions are translucent.

4. Add diced sweet potatoes, diced red and green bell peppers, ground turmeric, smoked paprika, salt, and pepper to the skillet. Sauté until the sweet potatoes are tender.

5. In a large bowl, mix together cooked quinoa and the sautéed vegetable mixture.

6. In a separate bowl, whisk together eggs and unsweetened almond milk.

7. Grease a baking dish and spread the quinoa and vegetable mixture evenly. Pour the egg and almond milk mixture over it.

8. Top the casserole with crumbled feta cheese.

9. Bake in the preheated oven for 30-35 minutes, or until the eggs are set.

10. Garnish with chopped fresh parsley before serving.

11. Allow the casserole to cool before storing it in meal prep containers. Store in the refrigerator for a heart-healthy, low-sodium, and anti-inflammatory meal prep option.

Nutritional Information (per serving):

- Carbs: 40g
- Sodium: 160mg
- Fats: 15g
- Protein: 12g

Cumin-Spiced Quinoa and Black Bean Bowl

Prep Time: 15 minutes | **Cook Time:** 25 minutes | **Servings:** 4

Ingredients:

- 1 cup quinoa, rinsed
- 2 cups low-sodium vegetable broth
- 1 can (15 ounces) black beans, drained and rinsed
- 1 cup corn kernels (fresh or frozen)
- 1 red bell pepper, diced
- 1 avocado, sliced
- 1/4 cup fresh cilantro, chopped
- 1 lime, juiced
- 1 tablespoon olive oil
- 1 teaspoon ground cumin
- 1/2 teaspoon smoked paprika
- 1/2 teaspoon garlic powder
- Salt and pepper to taste
- Optional toppings: Greek yogurt, salsa

Instructions:

1. In a medium saucepan, combine quinoa and low-sodium vegetable broth. Bring to a boil, then reduce heat to low, cover, and simmer for 15 minutes or until quinoa is cooked and liquid is absorbed. Fluff with a fork and let it cool.

2. In a large bowl, mix the cooked quinoa, black beans, corn kernels, diced red bell pepper, sliced avocado, and chopped fresh cilantro.

3. In a small bowl, whisk together lime juice, olive oil, ground cumin, smoked paprika, garlic powder, salt, and pepper.

4. Pour the dressing over the quinoa and black bean mixture. Toss gently to combine and ensure an even coating.

5. Divide the mixture into meal prep containers.

6. Optional: Top each serving with a dollop of Greek yogurt or salsa before serving.

7. Store in the refrigerator for a heart-healthy, low-sodium, and anti-inflammatory meal prep option.

Nutritional Information (per serving):

- Carbs: 45g
- Sodium: 180mg
- Fats: 15g
- Protein: 10g

Teriyaki Salmon and Quinoa Lettuce Wraps

Prep Time: 20 minutes | **Cook Time:** 15 minutes | **Servings:** 4

Ingredients:

- 1 cup quinoa, rinsed
- 2 cups low-sodium vegetable broth
- 4 salmon fillets
- 1/2 cup low-sodium teriyaki sauce
- 1 tablespoon olive oil
- 1 cup red cabbage, thinly sliced
- 1 carrot, julienned
- 1/2 cup cucumber, diced
- 1/4 cup green onions, sliced
- 1/4 cup fresh cilantro, chopped
- 1 tablespoon sesame seeds
- 1 head of butter lettuce leaves, washed and separated

Instructions:

1. In a medium saucepan, combine quinoa and low-sodium vegetable broth. Bring to a boil, then reduce heat to low, cover, and simmer for 15 minutes or until quinoa is cooked and liquid is absorbed. Fluff with a fork and let it cool.

2. Preheat the oven to 400°F (200°C).

3. Place salmon fillets on a baking sheet lined with parchment paper. Brush each fillet with low-sodium teriyaki sauce.

4. Bake in the preheated oven for 12-15 minutes or until the salmon is cooked through.

5. While the salmon is baking, heat olive oil in a skillet over medium heat. Add thinly sliced red cabbage, julienned carrots, diced cucumber, sliced green onions, and chopped fresh cilantro. Sauté until the vegetables are tender-crisp.

6. Fluff the cooled quinoa with a fork and add it to the skillet with the sautéed vegetables. Mix well to combine.

7. Once the salmon is cooked, flake it into bite-sized pieces with a fork.

8. To assemble the wraps, place a spoonful of quinoa and vegetable mixture onto a lettuce leaf. Top with flaked teriyaki salmon.

9. Sprinkle sesame seeds over each wrap.

10. Store the components separately in meal prep containers. Assemble wraps just before serving.

11. Store in the refrigerator for a heart-healthy, low-sodium, and anti-inflammatory meal prep option.

Nutritional Information (per serving):

- Carbs: 30g
- Sodium: 250mg
- Fats: 10g
- Protein: 25g

Grilled Vegetable and Quinoa Stuffed Portobello Mushrooms

Prep Time: 20 minutes | **Cook Time:** 20 minutes | **Servings:** 4

Ingredients:

- 4 large portobello mushrooms, stems removed
- 1 cup quinoa, rinsed
- 2 cups low-sodium vegetable broth
- 1 zucchini, sliced
- 1 yellow bell pepper, sliced
- 1 red onion, sliced
- 1 cup cherry tomatoes, halved
- 2 tablespoons olive oil
- 2 cloves garlic, minced
- 1 teaspoon dried thyme
- 1 teaspoon dried rosemary
- Salt and pepper to taste
- Fresh parsley, chopped (for garnish)

Instructions:

1. Preheat the grill to medium heat.

2. In a medium saucepan, combine quinoa and low-sodium vegetable broth. Bring to a boil, then reduce heat to low, cover, and simmer for 15 minutes or until quinoa is cooked and liquid is absorbed. Fluff with a fork and let it cool.

3. Brush portobello mushrooms with olive oil on both sides. Place them on the preheated grill, cap side down. Grill for 4-5 minutes on each side, or until mushrooms are tender.

4. While the mushrooms are grilling, in a large bowl, toss zucchini slices, yellow bell pepper slices, red onion slices, and halved cherry tomatoes with olive oil, minced garlic, dried thyme, dried rosemary, salt, and pepper.

5. Grill the vegetable mixture in a grill basket or on a skewer for about 5-7 minutes, or until the vegetables are tender and slightly charred.

6. In the same bowl as the vegetables, mix in the cooked quinoa.

7. Once the mushrooms are grilled, fill each cap with the quinoa and vegetable mixture.

8. Garnish with chopped fresh parsley.

9. Allow the stuffed mushrooms to cool before transferring them to meal prep containers. Store in the refrigerator for a heart-healthy, low-sodium, and anti-inflammatory meal prep option.

Nutritional Information (per serving):

- Carbs: 35g
- Sodium: 150mg
- Fats: 10g
- Protein: 8g

Quinoa and Chickpea Curry

Prep Time: 15 minutes | **Cook Time:** 30 minutes | **Servings:** 4

Ingredients:

- 1 cup quinoa, rinsed
- 2 cups low-sodium vegetable broth
- 1 can (15 ounces) chickpeas, drained and rinsed
- 1 onion, finely chopped
- 2 cloves garlic, minced
- 1 tablespoon olive oil
- 1 tablespoon curry powder
- 1 teaspoon ground turmeric
- 1 teaspoon ground cumin
- 1/2 teaspoon ground coriander
- 1/2 teaspoon paprika
- 1/2 teaspoon cayenne pepper (optional for heat)
- 1 can (14 ounces) diced tomatoes
- 1 can (14 ounces) coconut milk
- Salt and pepper to taste
- Fresh cilantro, chopped (for garnish)

Instructions:

1. In a medium saucepan, combine quinoa and low-sodium vegetable broth. Bring to a boil, then reduce heat to low, cover, and simmer for 15 minutes or until quinoa is cooked and liquid is absorbed. Fluff with a fork and let it cool.

2. In a large skillet, heat olive oil over medium heat. Add finely chopped onion and minced garlic. Sauté until the onions are translucent.

3. Add curry powder, ground turmeric, ground cumin, ground coriander, paprika, and cayenne pepper (if using) to the skillet. Stir to coat the onions and garlic with the spices.

4. Add drained and rinsed chickpeas to the skillet. Mix well.

5. Pour in diced tomatoes and coconut milk. Stir to combine.

6. Season with salt and pepper to taste. Simmer for 15-20 minutes, allowing the flavors to meld and the curry to thicken.

7. Fluff the cooled quinoa with a fork and add it to the curry mixture. Mix well.

8. Garnish with chopped fresh cilantro before serving.

9. Allow the curry to cool before transferring it to meal prep containers. Store in the refrigerator for a heart-healthy, low-sodium, and anti-inflammatory meal prep option.

Nutritional Information (per serving):

- Carbs: 45g
- Sodium: 200mg
- Fats: 15g
- Protein: 10g

Citrus-Marinated Shrimp and Quinoa Skewers

Prep Time: 20 minutes | **Marinating Time:** 30 minutes | **Cook Time:** 10 minutes | **Servings:** 4

Ingredients:

- 1 cup quinoa, rinsed
- 2 cups low-sodium vegetable broth
- 1 pound large shrimp, peeled and deveined
- Zest and juice of 1 lemon
- Zest and juice of 1 orange
- 2 tablespoons olive oil
- 2 cloves garlic, minced
- 1 teaspoon ground cumin
- 1 teaspoon paprika
- 1/2 teaspoon ground coriander
- Salt and pepper to taste
- 1 red bell pepper, diced
- 1 yellow bell pepper, diced
- 1 zucchini, sliced
- Wooden skewers, soaked in water

Instructions:

1. In a medium saucepan, combine quinoa and low-sodium vegetable broth. Bring to a boil, then reduce heat to low, cover, and simmer for 15 minutes or until quinoa is cooked and liquid is absorbed. Fluff with a fork and let it cool.

2. In a bowl, combine the peeled and deveined shrimp with lemon zest, lemon juice, orange zest, orange juice, olive oil, minced garlic, ground cumin, paprika, ground coriander, salt, and pepper. Allow the shrimp to marinate for at least 30 minutes.

3. Preheat the grill or grill pan over medium-high heat.

4. Thread the marinated shrimp, diced red bell pepper, diced yellow bell pepper, and sliced zucchini onto the soaked wooden skewers.

5. Grill the skewers for about 3-4 minutes on each side or until the shrimp are opaque and cooked through.

6. While the skewers are grilling, fluff the cooled quinoa with a fork.

7. Serve the grilled shrimp and vegetable skewers over a bed of quinoa.

8. Allow the skewers to cool before storing them in meal prep containers. Store in the refrigerator for a heart-healthy, low-sodium, and anti-inflammatory meal prep option.

Nutritional Information (per serving):

- Carbs: 35g
- Sodium: 180mg
- Fats: 8g
- Protein: 25g

Tomato and Basil Quinoa Risotto

Prep Time: 15 minutes | **Cook Time:** 25 minutes | **Servings:** 4

Ingredients:

- 1 cup quinoa, rinsed
- 2 cups low-sodium vegetable broth
- 2 tablespoons olive oil
- 1 onion, finely chopped
- 2 cloves garlic, minced
- 1 can (14 ounces) diced tomatoes
- 1 teaspoon dried basil
- 1/2 teaspoon dried oregano
- 1/2 teaspoon dried thyme
- Salt and pepper to taste
- 1/4 cup fresh basil, chopped (for garnish)
- Grated Parmesan cheese (optional, for serving)

Instructions:

1. In a medium saucepan, combine quinoa and low-sodium vegetable broth. Bring to a boil, then reduce heat to low, cover, and simmer for 15 minutes or until quinoa is cooked and liquid is absorbed. Fluff with a fork and let it cool.

2. In a large skillet, heat olive oil over medium heat. Add finely chopped onion and minced garlic. Sauté until the onions are translucent.

3. Add the can of diced tomatoes (including juice) to the skillet. Stir in dried basil, dried oregano, dried thyme, salt, and pepper.

4. Simmer the tomato mixture for 10-15 minutes, allowing the flavors to meld and the tomatoes to break down.

5. Fluff the cooled quinoa with a fork and add it to the skillet with the tomato mixture. Mix well.

6. Allow the risotto to simmer for an additional 5-7 minutes, ensuring the quinoa is well coated and heated through.

7. Garnish the risotto with chopped fresh basil.

8. Optional: Serve with a sprinkle of grated Parmesan cheese.

9. Allow the risotto to cool before transferring it to meal prep containers. Store in the refrigerator for a heart-healthy, low-sodium, and anti-inflammatory meal prep option.

Nutritional Information (per serving):

- Carbs: 40g
- Sodium: 150mg
- Fats: 8g
- Protein: 10g

Quinoa and Edamame Salad with Miso Dressing

Prep Time: 20 minutes | **Cook Time:** 15 minutes | **Servings:** 4

Ingredients:

For the Salad:

- 1 cup quinoa, rinsed
- 2 cups water
- 1 cup edamame, shelled

For the Miso Dressing:

- 3 tablespoons white miso paste
- 2 tablespoons rice vinegar
- 1 tablespoon sesame oil
- 1 tablespoon soy sauce (low-sodium)

- 1 red bell pepper, diced
- 1 carrot, julienned
- 1/4 cup green onions, sliced
- 1/4 cup fresh cilantro, chopped
- 1 tablespoon honey or maple syrup
- 1 teaspoon fresh ginger, grated
- 1 clove garlic, minced
- 2 tablespoons water

Instructions:

1. In a medium saucepan, combine quinoa and water. Bring to a boil, then reduce heat to low, cover, and simmer for 15 minutes or until quinoa is cooked and liquid is absorbed. Fluff with a fork and let it cool.

2. In a small saucepan, bring water to a boil. Add shelled edamame and cook for 3-5 minutes. Drain and set aside.

3. In a large bowl, combine cooked quinoa, boiled edamame, diced red bell pepper, julienned carrot, sliced green onions, and chopped fresh cilantro.

4. In a separate bowl, whisk together white miso paste, rice vinegar, sesame oil, low-sodium soy sauce, honey (or maple syrup), grated fresh ginger, minced garlic, and water. Adjust the consistency by adding more water if needed.

5. Pour the miso dressing over the quinoa and vegetable mixture. Toss gently to coat the salad evenly.

6. Allow the salad to chill in the refrigerator for at least 30 minutes to let the flavors meld.

7. Portion the salad into meal prep containers for a heart-healthy, low-sodium, and anti-inflammatory meal prep option.

Nutritional Information (per serving):

- Carbs: 40g
- Sodium: 250mg
- Fats: 10g
- Protein: 12g

<u>Roasted Garlic and Herb Quinoa Patties</u>

Prep Time: 20 minutes | **Cook Time:** 25 minutes | **Servings:** 4

Ingredients:

- 1 cup quinoa, rinsed
- 2 cups low-sodium vegetable broth
- 1 bulb of garlic
- 2 tablespoons olive oil, divided
- 1/2 cup breadcrumbs (whole grain for added health benefits)
- 1/4 cup grated Parmesan cheese
- 1/4 cup fresh parsley, chopped
- 2 teaspoons dried oregano
- 1 teaspoon dried thyme
- Salt and pepper to taste
- 2 eggs, beaten
- Cooking spray

Instructions:

1. In a medium saucepan, combine quinoa and low-sodium vegetable broth. Bring to a boil, then reduce heat to low, cover, and simmer for 15 minutes or until quinoa is cooked and liquid is absorbed. Fluff with a fork and let it cool.

2. Preheat the oven to 400°F (200°C).

3. Cut the top off the bulb of garlic to expose the cloves. Place it on a piece of foil, drizzle with 1 tablespoon of olive oil, and wrap it tightly. Roast in the preheated oven for about 20-25 minutes or until the garlic is soft and golden. Allow it to cool.

4. In a large bowl, combine the cooked quinoa, breadcrumbs, grated Parmesan cheese, chopped fresh parsley, dried oregano, dried thyme, salt, and pepper.

5. Squeeze the roasted garlic cloves out of their skins into the quinoa mixture. Mix well.

6. Add beaten eggs to the quinoa mixture and stir until the mixture is well combined.

7. Form the mixture into patties. Use your hands to shape them, ensuring they hold together.

8. Heat the remaining 1 tablespoon of olive oil in a skillet over medium heat. Place the quinoa patties in the skillet and cook for 4-5 minutes on each side or until they are golden brown and cooked through.

9. Allow the patties to cool before transferring them to meal prep containers. Store in the refrigerator for a heart-healthy, low-sodium, and anti-inflammatory meal prep option.

Nutritional Information (per serving):

- Carbs: 30g
- Sodium: 180mg
- Fats: 12g
- Protein: 10g

Chapter 5: Lean Protein Dishes

Baked Turmeric Chicken Thighs with Brussels Sprouts

Prep Time: 15 minutes | **Cook Time:** 40 minutes | **Servings:** 4

Ingredients:

- 4 bone-in, skin-on chicken thighs
- 1 pound Brussels sprouts, halved
- 3 tablespoons olive oil
- 2 teaspoons ground turmeric
- 1 teaspoon garlic powder
- 1 teaspoon onion powder
- 1 teaspoon paprika
- 1/2 teaspoon black pepper
- 1/2 teaspoon sea salt
- 1 lemon, sliced

Instructions:

1. Preheat the oven to 400°F (200°C).
2. Pat dry the chicken thighs with paper towels.
3. In a small bowl, mix turmeric, garlic powder, onion powder, paprika, black pepper, and sea salt.
4. Rub the spice mixture evenly over the chicken thighs.
5. In a large bowl, toss the halved Brussels sprouts with 2 tablespoons of olive oil.
6. Season with a pinch of salt and pepper.
7. Arrange the seasoned chicken thighs and Brussels sprouts in a single layer in a baking dish.
8. Place lemon slices over the chicken.
9. Drizzle the remaining 1 tablespoon of olive oil over the chicken and Brussels sprouts.
10. Bake in the preheated oven for 40 minutes or until the chicken reaches an internal temperature of 165°F (74°C).
11. Once baked, let it rest for a few minutes before serving.
12. For meal prep, divide the chicken and Brussels sprouts into separate containers.

Nutritional Information (per serving):

- **Carbs:** 15g
- **Sodium:** 400mg
- **Fats:** 20g
- **Protein:** 25g

Ginger-Soy Glazed Salmon with Asparagus

Prep Time: 15 minutes | **Cook Time:** 15 minutes | **Servings:** 4

Ingredients:

- 4 salmon fillets
- 1 pound asparagus, ends trimmed
- 3 tablespoons low-sodium soy sauce
- 2 tablespoons honey
- 1 tablespoon grated fresh ginger
- 2 cloves garlic, minced
- 1 tablespoon olive oil
- 1/2 teaspoon ground black pepper
- Sesame seeds and chopped green onions for garnish

Instructions:

1. Preheat the oven to 400°F (200°C).
2. In a small bowl, whisk together soy sauce, honey, grated ginger, minced garlic, and black pepper.
3. Place the salmon fillets in a shallow dish and pour half of the ginger-soy glaze over them. Let it marinate for 10 minutes.
4. Lay the trimmed asparagus on a baking sheet.
5. Drizzle with olive oil and season with a pinch of black pepper.
6. Place marinated salmon fillets on the same baking sheet with asparagus.
7. Bake for 12-15 minutes or until the salmon is cooked through and flakes easily with a fork.
8. In the last 5 minutes of baking, brush the remaining ginger-soy glaze over the salmon.
9. Garnish with sesame seeds and chopped green onions.
10. Serve immediately or allow it to cool before storing in meal prep containers.

Nutritional Information (per serving):

- **Carbs:** 15g
- **Sodium:** 300mg
- **Fats:** 12g
- **Protein:** 30g

Lemon-Herb Grilled Turkey Breast

Prep Time: 20 minutes | **Cook Time:** 30 minutes | **Servings:** 6

Ingredients:

- 1.5 pounds turkey breast, boneless and skinless
- 3 tablespoons olive oil
- 2 tablespoons fresh lemon juice
- 2 teaspoons dried thyme
- 2 teaspoons dried rosemary
- 1 teaspoon garlic powder
- 1 teaspoon onion powder
- 1/2 teaspoon paprika
- Salt and black pepper to taste
- Fresh parsley for garnish

Instructions:

1. Preheat the grill to medium-high heat.
2. In a small bowl, whisk together olive oil, lemon juice, dried thyme, dried rosemary, garlic powder, onion powder, paprika, salt, and black pepper.
3. Place the turkey breast in a shallow dish and coat it evenly with the lemon-herb marinade. Allow it to marinate for at least 15 minutes.
4. Grill the turkey breast for approximately 15 minutes per side or until the internal temperature reaches 165°F (74°C).
5. While grilling, baste the turkey with the remaining marinade to keep it moist and flavorful.
6. Allow the grilled turkey breast to rest for a few minutes before slicing it into thin, even slices.
7. Garnish with fresh parsley before serving.
8. Serve immediately or let it cool before storing in meal prep containers.

Nutritional Information (per serving):

- **Carbs:** 1g
- **Sodium:** 200mg
- **Fats:** 8g
- **Protein:** 30g

<u>Chili-Lime Tofu and Broccoli Stir-Fry</u>

Prep Time: 15 minutes | **Cook Time:** 15 minutes | **Servings:** 4

Ingredients:

- 1 block (14 ounces) extra-firm tofu, pressed and cubed
- 4 cups broccoli florets
- 3 tablespoons low-sodium soy sauce
- 2 tablespoons lime juice
- 1 tablespoon maple syrup
- 1 teaspoon chili powder
- 1 teaspoon ground cumin
- 1/2 teaspoon turmeric powder
- 2 tablespoons sesame oil
- 3 cloves garlic, minced
- 1 tablespoon grated fresh ginger
- Brown rice or quinoa for serving
- Sesame seeds and sliced green onions for garnish

Instructions:

1. Press the tofu to remove excess water, then cut it into cubes.
2. In a small bowl, whisk together soy sauce, lime juice, maple syrup, chili powder, ground cumin, and turmeric powder to create the sauce.
3. Toss the tofu cubes in half of the prepared sauce and let them marinate for at least 10 minutes.
4. In a large skillet or wok, heat sesame oil over medium-high heat.
5. Add marinated tofu cubes and stir-fry until they are golden brown and crisp. Set aside.
6. In the same skillet, add a bit more sesame oil if needed.
7. Add minced garlic and grated ginger, and stir for a minute.
8. Add broccoli florets and stir-fry until they are tender-crisp.
9. Return the cooked tofu to the skillet with broccoli, and pour the remaining sauce over the mixture.
10. Toss everything together until well-coated and heated through.
11. Serve the stir-fry over brown rice or quinoa.
12. Garnish with sesame seeds and sliced green onions.
13. Allow to cool before storing in meal prep containers.

Nutritional Information (per serving):

- **Carbs:** 20g
- **Sodium:** 300mg
- **Fats:** 12g
- **Protein:** 15g

Oven-Roasted Cod with Tomato-Olive Relish

Prep Time: 15 minutes | **Cook Time:** 20 minutes | **Servings:** 4

Ingredients:

For Cod:

- 4 cod fillets (about 6 ounces each)
- 2 tablespoons olive oil
- 1 teaspoon dried oregano

For Tomato-Olive Relish:

- 1 cup cherry tomatoes, halved
- 1/2 cup Kalamata olives, sliced
- 1/4 cup red onion, finely chopped

- 1 teaspoon paprika
- 1/2 teaspoon garlic powder
- 1/2 teaspoon onion powder
- Salt and black pepper to taste
- 2 tablespoons fresh parsley, chopped
- 1 tablespoon olive oil
- 1 tablespoon red wine vinegar
- Salt and black pepper to taste

Instructions:

1. Preheat the oven to 400°F (200°C).
2. Place cod fillets on a baking sheet lined with parchment paper.
3. In a small bowl, mix olive oil, dried oregano, paprika, garlic powder, onion powder, salt, and black pepper.
4. Rub the spice mixture evenly over each cod fillet.
5. Roast the cod in the preheated oven for 15-20 minutes or until the fish flakes easily with a fork.
6. In a medium bowl, combine halved cherry tomatoes, sliced Kalamata olives, chopped red onion, and fresh parsley.
7. In a small bowl, whisk together olive oil, red wine vinegar, salt, and black pepper.
8. Pour the dressing over the tomato-olive mixture and toss to combine.
9. Spoon the tomato-olive relish over the roasted cod fillets.
10. Garnish with additional fresh parsley.
11. Allow to cool before storing in meal prep containers.

Nutritional Information (per serving):

- **Carbs:** 5g
- **Sodium:** 300mg
- **Fats:** 10g
- **Protein:** 30g

Green Tea Poached Chicken with Bok Choy

Prep Time: 15 minutes | **Cook Time:** 25 minutes | **Servings:** 4

Ingredients:

For Green Tea Poached Chicken:

- 4 boneless, skinless chicken breasts
- 4 green tea bags
- 4 cups hot water
- 3 slices fresh ginger

For Bok Choy:

- 4 baby bok choy, halved
- 1 tablespoon olive oil
- 2 cloves garlic, minced

- 2 cloves garlic, smashed
- 1 tablespoon low-sodium soy sauce
- 1 tablespoon honey
- 1 teaspoon sesame oil

- 1 teaspoon fresh ginger, grated
- 1 tablespoon low-sodium soy sauce
- 1 tablespoon rice vinegar

Instructions:

1. In a large pot, steep the green tea bags in hot water to create a tea broth.
2. Add ginger, smashed garlic, low-sodium soy sauce, honey, and sesame oil to the tea broth.
3. Place the chicken breasts in the pot and simmer for 20-25 minutes until cooked through.
4. While the chicken is poaching, heat olive oil in a skillet over medium heat.
5. Add minced garlic and grated ginger to the skillet, sautéing until fragrant.
6. Add halved baby bok choy, low-sodium soy sauce, and rice vinegar. Sauté until bok choy is tender-crisp.
7. Once the chicken is cooked, remove from the tea broth.
8. Serve the poached chicken on a bed of sautéed bok choy.
9. Strain the tea broth to remove solids, creating a clear broth.
10. Serve the green tea broth alongside the chicken and bok choy.
11. Garnish with fresh herbs if desired.
12. Allow to cool before storing chicken, bok choy, and broth in meal prep containers.

Nutritional Information (per serving):

- **Carbs:** 8g
- **Sodium:** 200mg
- **Fats:** 5g
- **Protein:** 30g

Pesto-Marinated Grilled Shrimp Skewers

Prep Time: 20 minutes | **Cook Time:** 8 minutes | **Servings:** 4

Ingredients:

- 1 pound large shrimp, peeled and deveined
- 1/2 cup fresh basil leaves
- 1/4 cup pine nuts, toasted
- 2 cloves garlic, minced
- 1/4 cup extra-virgin olive oil
- 1 tablespoon lemon juice
- 1/4 teaspoon red pepper flakes (optional)
- Salt and black pepper to taste
- Wooden skewers, soaked in water

Instructions:

1. In a food processor, combine fresh basil leaves, toasted pine nuts, minced garlic, extra-virgin olive oil, lemon juice, red pepper flakes (if using), salt, and black pepper. Blend until a smooth pesto marinade is formed.
2. Place the peeled and deveined shrimp in a bowl.
3. Coat the shrimp with the pesto marinade, ensuring each shrimp is well-covered.
4. Allow the shrimp to marinate for at least 15 minutes.
5. Preheat the grill to medium-high heat.
6. Thread the marinated shrimp onto soaked wooden skewers, distributing them evenly.
7. Grill the shrimp skewers for approximately 3-4 minutes per side or until the shrimp turn pink and opaque.
8. Serve the grilled shrimp skewers immediately or let them cool before storing in meal prep containers.

Nutritional Information (per serving):

- **Carbs:** 2g
- **Sodium:** 150mg
- **Fats:** 15g
- **Protein:** 25g

Cilantro-Lime Chicken and Avocado Salad

Prep Time: 15 minutes | **Cook Time:** 15 minutes | **Servings:** 4

Ingredients:

For Cilantro-Lime Chicken:

- 4 boneless, skinless chicken breasts
- 2 tablespoons olive oil
- 3 cloves garlic, minced
- 1 teaspoon ground cumin
- 1 teaspoon smoked paprika
- 1/2 teaspoon chili powder
- Zest and juice of 2 limes
- Salt and black pepper to taste

For Salad:

- 6 cups mixed salad greens
- 2 avocados, sliced
- 1 cup cherry tomatoes, halved
- 1/2 red onion, thinly sliced
- 1/4 cup fresh cilantro leaves

For Dressing:

- 3 tablespoons olive oil
- Zest and juice of 1 lime
- 1 teaspoon honey
- Salt and black pepper to taste

Instructions:

1. In a bowl, mix olive oil, minced garlic, ground cumin, smoked paprika, chili powder, lime zest, lime juice, salt, and black pepper.
2. Coat the chicken breasts with the marinade and let them marinate for at least 15 minutes.
3. Grill or pan-cook the chicken until fully cooked. Once done, let it rest for a few minutes before slicing.
4. In a large bowl, toss mixed salad greens, sliced avocados, halved cherry tomatoes, thinly sliced red onion, and fresh cilantro leaves.
5. In a small bowl, whisk together olive oil, lime zest, lime juice, honey, salt, and black pepper to create the dressing.
6. Drizzle the dressing over the salad and toss until all ingredients are well-coated.
7. Top the salad with sliced cilantro-lime chicken.
8. Serve immediately or let it cool before storing in meal prep containers.

Nutritional Information (per serving):

- **Carbs:** 15g
- **Sodium:** 200mg
- **Fats:** 20g
- **Protein:** 30g

<u>Miso-Glazed Sea Bass with Sesame Green Beans</u>

Prep Time: 20 minutes | **Cook Time:** 15 minutes | **Servings:** 4

Ingredients:

For Miso-Glazed Sea Bass:

- 4 sea bass fillets (6 ounces each)
- 3 tablespoons white miso paste
- 2 tablespoons mirin
- 1 tablespoon low-sodium soy sauce

For Sesame Green Beans:

- 1 pound green beans, trimmed
- 1 tablespoon sesame oil

- 1 tablespoon honey
- 1 tablespoon sesame oil
- 2 cloves garlic, minced
- 1 tablespoon grated fresh ginger
- Sesame seeds for garnish
- 1 tablespoon low-sodium soy sauce
- 1 tablespoon sesame seeds

Instructions:

1. Preheat the oven to 400°F (200°C).
2. In a bowl, whisk together white miso paste, mirin, low-sodium soy sauce, honey, sesame oil, minced garlic, and grated fresh ginger.
3. Place sea bass fillets on a baking sheet lined with parchment paper.
4. Spread the miso glaze over each sea bass fillet.
5. Bake in the preheated oven for 12-15 minutes or until the sea bass is cooked through and flakes easily with a fork.
6. Garnish with sesame seeds.
7. In a large skillet, heat sesame oil over medium heat.
8. Add trimmed green beans and sauté until they are tender-crisp.
9. Drizzle low-sodium soy sauce over the green beans and sprinkle sesame seeds. Toss to coat.
10. Serve the miso-glazed sea bass over sesame green beans.
11. Allow to cool before storing in meal prep containers.

Nutritional Information (per serving):

- **Carbs:** 10g
- **Sodium:** 300mg
- **Fats:** 15g
- **Protein:** 30g

Rosemary-Dijon Baked Pork Chops with Cauliflower Mash

Prep Time: 20 minutes | **Cook Time:** 30 minutes | **Servings:** 4

Ingredients:

For Baked Pork Chops:

- 4 bone-in pork chops
- 2 tablespoons Dijon mustard
- 1 tablespoon olive oil

For Cauliflower Mash:

- 1 large head cauliflower, chopped
- 2 tablespoons olive oil
- 2 cloves garlic, minced

- 2 cloves garlic, minced
- 1 tablespoon fresh rosemary, chopped
- Salt and black pepper to taste

- 1/4 cup unsweetened almond milk
- Salt and black pepper to taste
- Chopped fresh chives for garnish

Instructions:

1. Preheat the oven to 400°F (200°C).
2. In a small bowl, mix Dijon mustard, olive oil, minced garlic, chopped fresh rosemary, salt, and black pepper.
3. Pat dry the pork chops and rub the Dijon mixture over each pork chop, coating them evenly.
4. Place the pork chops on a baking sheet.
5. Bake in the preheated oven for 25-30 minutes or until the pork chops reach an internal temperature of 145°F (63°C).
6. Steam the chopped cauliflower until tender.
7. In a skillet, heat olive oil over medium heat.
8. Add minced garlic and sauté until fragrant.
9. Add steamed cauliflower to the skillet and mash with a fork or potato masher.
10. Stir in unsweetened almond milk and continue mashing until desired consistency is reached.
11. Season with salt and black pepper to taste.
12. Serve the rosemary-Dijon baked pork chops over cauliflower mash.
13. Garnish with chopped fresh chives.
14. Allow to cool before storing in meal prep containers.

Nutritional Information (per serving):

- **Carbs:** 10g
- **Sodium:** 200mg

- **Fats:** 15g
- **Protein:** 30g

<u>Spicy Ginger-Orange Glazed Tempeh</u>

Prep Time: 15 minutes | **Cook Time:** 20 minutes | **Servings:** 4

Ingredients:

- 2 packages (about 16 ounces) tempeh, sliced
- 1/4 cup low-sodium soy sauce
- 1/4 cup orange juice
- 2 tablespoons rice vinegar
- 2 tablespoons fresh ginger, grated
- 2 cloves garlic, minced
- 2 tablespoons maple syrup
- 1 tablespoon sesame oil
- 1/2 teaspoon red pepper flakes (adjust to taste)
- 2 tablespoons olive oil
- Sesame seeds and sliced green onions for garnish

Instructions:

1. Steam tempeh slices for 10 minutes to reduce bitterness. Allow them to cool.
2. In a bowl, whisk together low-sodium soy sauce, orange juice, rice vinegar, grated fresh ginger, minced garlic, maple syrup, sesame oil, and red pepper flakes.
3. Place the cooled tempeh slices in a shallow dish and pour half of the glaze over them. Let it marinate for at least 15 minutes.
4. In a skillet, heat olive oil over medium-high heat.
5. Add marinated tempeh slices to the skillet and cook until golden brown on both sides.
6. Pour the remaining glaze over the tempeh slices, ensuring they are well-coated.
7. Allow the glaze to thicken for a few minutes.
8. Serve the spicy ginger-orange glazed tempeh over a bed of rice or quinoa.
9. Garnish with sesame seeds and sliced green onions.
10. Allow to cool before storing in meal prep containers.

Nutritional Information (per serving):

- **Carbs:** 15g
- **Sodium:** 250mg
- **Fats:** 12g
- **Protein:** 20g

Herb-Crusted Mahi-Mahi with Roasted Vegetables

Prep Time: 15 minutes | **Cook Time:** 25 minutes | **Servings:** 4

Ingredients:

For Mahi-Mahi:

- 4 mahi-mahi fillets (6 ounces each)
- 2 tablespoons olive oil
- 2 tablespoons Dijon mustard
- 2 cloves garlic, minced

- 1 tablespoon fresh parsley, chopped
- 1 tablespoon fresh thyme leaves
- 1 teaspoon lemon zest
- Salt and black pepper to taste

For Roasted Vegetables:

- 1 pound baby potatoes, halved
- 2 cups baby carrots
- 1 red bell pepper, sliced
- 1 yellow bell pepper, sliced

- 1 zucchini, sliced
- 2 tablespoons olive oil
- 1 teaspoon dried rosemary
- 1 teaspoon dried oregano
- Salt and black pepper to taste

Instructions:

1. Preheat the oven to 400°F (200°C).
2. In a bowl, mix olive oil, Dijon mustard, minced garlic, chopped fresh parsley, fresh thyme leaves, lemon zest, salt, and black pepper.
3. Pat dry the mahi-mahi fillets and coat them with the herb mixture.
4. In a large mixing bowl, combine halved baby potatoes, baby carrots, sliced red bell pepper, sliced yellow bell pepper, and sliced zucchini.
5. Drizzle olive oil over the vegetables and sprinkle dried rosemary, dried oregano, salt, and black pepper. Toss until well-coated.
6. Place the herb-crusted mahi-mahi fillets on one side of a baking sheet and the prepared vegetables on the other side.
7. Roast in the preheated oven for 20-25 minutes or until the fish is cooked through and the vegetables are tender.
8. Serve the herb-crusted mahi-mahi fillets with a side of roasted vegetables.
9. Allow to cool before storing in meal prep containers.

Nutritional Information (per serving):

- **Carbs:** 25g
- **Sodium:** 250mg
- **Fats:** 10g
- **Protein:** 30g

Harissa-Marinated Lamb Kebabs with Quinoa Tabouleh

Prep Time: 30 minutes | **Cook Time:** 15 minutes | **Servings:** 4

Ingredients:

For Lamb Kebabs:

- 1.5 pounds lamb leg meat, cubed
- 3 tablespoons harissa paste
- 2 tablespoons olive oil
- 2 cloves garlic, minced

For Quinoa Tabouleh:

- 1 cup quinoa, rinsed and cooked
- 1 cucumber, finely diced
- 1 cup cherry tomatoes, diced
- 1/2 red onion, finely chopped

- 1 teaspoon ground cumin
- 1 teaspoon ground coriander
- Salt and black pepper to taste
- Wooden skewers, soaked in water

- 1 cup fresh parsley, chopped
- 1/2 cup fresh mint, chopped
- 1/4 cup olive oil
- Zest and juice of 1 lemon
- Salt and black pepper to taste

Instructions:

1. In a bowl, combine cubed lamb leg meat, harissa paste, olive oil, minced garlic, ground cumin, ground coriander, salt, and black pepper.
2. Allow the lamb to marinate for at least 20 minutes.
3. In a large bowl, combine cooked quinoa, finely diced cucumber, diced cherry tomatoes, finely chopped red onion, chopped fresh parsley, and chopped fresh mint.
4. In a small bowl, whisk together olive oil, zest, and juice of 1 lemon, salt, and black pepper.
5. Pour the dressing over the quinoa mixture and toss until well combined.
6. Thread the marinated lamb cubes onto soaked wooden skewers.
7. Grill the lamb kebabs over medium-high heat for about 12-15 minutes or until cooked to your liking.
8. Serve the harissa-marinated lamb kebabs over a bed of quinoa tabouleh.
9. Garnish with extra fresh herbs if desired.
10. Allow to cool before storing lamb kebabs and quinoa tabouleh in meal prep containers.

Nutritional Information (per serving):

- **Carbs:** 30g
- **Sodium:** 200mg
- **Fats:** 15g

- **Protein:** 25g

Walnut-Crusted Chicken Tenders with Zucchini Noodles

Prep Time: 20 minutes | **Cook Time:** 15 minutes | **Servings:** 4

Ingredients:

For Walnut-Crusted Chicken Tenders:

- 1.5 pounds chicken tenders
- 1 cup walnuts, finely chopped
- 1/2 cup whole wheat flour
- 2 eggs, beaten

For Zucchini Noodles:

- 4 large zucchinis, spiralized
- 2 tablespoons olive oil
- 3 cloves garlic, minced

- 1 teaspoon dried thyme
- 1 teaspoon smoked paprika
- Salt and black pepper to taste
- Olive oil for cooking

- 1 teaspoon dried basil
- 1/2 teaspoon red pepper flakes (optional)
- Salt and black pepper to taste

Instructions:

1. In a shallow bowl, combine finely chopped walnuts, whole wheat flour, dried thyme, smoked paprika, salt, and black pepper.
2. Dip each chicken tender into beaten eggs, then coat with the walnut mixture, pressing the coating to adhere.
3. In a large skillet, heat olive oil over medium heat.
4. Cook the walnut-crusted chicken tenders for about 4-5 minutes per side or until golden brown and cooked through.
5. In a separate skillet, heat olive oil over medium heat.
6. Add minced garlic and sauté until fragrant.
7. Add spiralized zucchini, dried basil, red pepper flakes (if using), salt, and black pepper. Sauté until zucchini noodles are tender-crisp.
8. Serve the walnut-crusted chicken tenders over a bed of zucchini noodles.
9. Garnish with additional fresh herbs if desired.
10. Allow to cool before storing chicken tenders and zucchini noodles in meal prep containers.

Nutritional Information (per serving):

- **Carbs:** 15g
- **Sodium:** 300mg
- **Fats:** 20g
- **Protein:** 30g

Blackened Tilapia with Mango-Avocado Salsa

Prep Time: 20 minutes | **Cook Time:** 10 minutes | **Servings:** 4

Ingredients:

For Blackened Tilapia:

- 4 tilapia fillets
- 2 teaspoons paprika
- 1 teaspoon onion powder
- 1 teaspoon garlic powder
- 1 teaspoon dried thyme
- 1/2 teaspoon cayenne pepper
- 1/2 teaspoon black pepper
- 1/2 teaspoon dried oregano
- 1/2 teaspoon smoked paprika
- 1/4 teaspoon salt
- 2 tablespoons olive oil

For Mango-Avocado Salsa:

- 1 mango, diced
- 1 avocado, diced
- 1/2 red onion, finely chopped
- 1 jalapeño, seeded and finely diced
- 1/4 cup fresh cilantro, chopped
- Juice of 2 limes
- Salt and black pepper to taste

Instructions:

1. In a small bowl, mix paprika, onion powder, garlic powder, dried thyme, cayenne pepper, black pepper, dried oregano, smoked paprika, and salt.
2. Pat dry tilapia fillets and rub the spice mixture evenly on both sides.
3. Heat olive oil in a skillet over medium-high heat.
4. Cook the blackened tilapia fillets for about 3-4 minutes per side or until they are opaque and easily flake with a fork.
5. In a bowl, combine diced mango, diced avocado, finely chopped red onion, finely diced jalapeño, chopped fresh cilantro, lime juice, salt, and black pepper. Toss gently.
6. Serve the blackened tilapia fillets topped with mango-avocado salsa.
7. Garnish with additional cilantro if desired.
8. Allow to cool before storing blackened tilapia and mango-avocado salsa in meal prep containers.

Nutritional Information (per serving):

- **Carbs:** 15g
- **Sodium:** 250mg
- **Fats:** 10g
- **Protein:** 25g

Tandoori-Style Chicken Skewers with Cucumber Raita

Prep Time: 30 minutes | **Cook Time:** 15 minutes | **Servings:** 4

Ingredients:

For Tandoori-Style Chicken Skewers:

- 1.5 pounds chicken breasts, cut into cubes
- 1 cup plain Greek yogurt
- 2 tablespoons olive oil
- 2 teaspoons ground cumin
- 2 teaspoons ground coriander
- 1 teaspoon ground turmeric
- 1 teaspoon paprika
- 1 teaspoon cayenne pepper
- 2 teaspoons garam masala
- 4 cloves garlic, minced
- 1 tablespoon grated fresh ginger
- Salt and black pepper to taste
- Wooden skewers, soaked in water

For Cucumber Raita:

- 1 cucumber, grated
- 1 cup plain Greek yogurt
- 1 clove garlic, minced
- 1 tablespoon fresh mint, chopped
- 1 tablespoon fresh cilantro, chopped
- 1/2 teaspoon ground cumin
- Salt and black pepper to taste

Instructions:

1. In a bowl, mix together Greek yogurt, olive oil, ground cumin, ground coriander, ground turmeric, paprika, cayenne pepper, garam masala, minced garlic, grated fresh ginger, salt, and black pepper.
2. Add chicken cubes to the marinade, ensuring they are well-coated. Marinate for at least 2 hours or overnight.
3. Thread marinated chicken onto soaked wooden skewers.
4. Preheat the grill or grill pan over medium-high heat.
5. Grill the tandoori-style chicken skewers for about 6-8 minutes per side or until fully cooked.
6. In a bowl, combine grated cucumber, Greek yogurt, minced garlic, chopped fresh mint, chopped fresh cilantro, ground cumin, salt, and black pepper. Mix well.
7. Serve the tandoori-style chicken skewers with a side of cucumber raita.
8. Garnish with additional fresh herbs if desired.
9. Allow to cool before storing chicken skewers and cucumber raita in meal prep containers.

Nutritional Information (per serving):

- **Carbs:** 10g
- **Sodium:** 200mg
- **Fats:** 8g
- **Protein:** 30g

Sesame-Crusted Ahi Tuna with Spinach Salad

Prep Time: 15 minutes | **Cook Time:** 5 minutes | **Servings:** 4

Ingredients:

For Sesame-Crusted Ahi Tuna:

- 4 ahi tuna steaks (6 ounces each)
- 1/4 cup black sesame seeds
- 1/4 cup white sesame seeds
- 2 tablespoons soy sauce
- 1 tablespoon sesame oil
- 1 tablespoon honey
- 1 teaspoon grated fresh ginger
- 1 teaspoon minced garlic
- 1 tablespoon olive oil (for searing)

For Spinach Salad:

- 6 cups fresh spinach leaves
- 1 cup cherry tomatoes, halved
- 1 cucumber, thinly sliced
- 1/4 red onion, thinly sliced
- 1/4 cup extra virgin olive oil
- 2 tablespoons balsamic vinegar
- Salt and black pepper to taste

Instructions:

1. In a shallow dish, mix black sesame seeds and white sesame seeds.
2. In a separate bowl, whisk together soy sauce, sesame oil, honey, grated fresh ginger, and minced garlic.
3. Press each ahi tuna steak into the sesame seed mixture, coating both sides.
4. Heat olive oil in a skillet over high heat. Sear the sesame-crusted ahi tuna for about 1-2 minutes per side or until the sesame seeds are golden. The tuna should remain rare in the center.
5. In a large bowl, combine fresh spinach leaves, cherry tomatoes, thinly sliced cucumber, and thinly sliced red onion.
6. In a small bowl, whisk together extra virgin olive oil, balsamic vinegar, salt, and black pepper. Drizzle the dressing over the salad and toss gently to coat.
7. Serve the sesame-crusted ahi tuna over a bed of spinach salad.
8. Garnish with additional sesame seeds if desired.
9. Allow to cool before storing sesame-crusted ahi tuna and spinach salad in meal prep containers.

Nutritional Information (per serving):

- **Carbs:** 15g
- **Sodium:** 300mg
- **Fats:** 20g
- **Protein:** 30g

Greek Yogurt Marinated Chicken Kabobs with Tzatziki

Prep Time: 30 minutes | **Marinating Time:** 2 hours | **Cook Time:** 15 minutes | **Servings:** 4

Ingredients:

For Greek Yogurt Marinated Chicken:

- 1.5 pounds chicken breast, cut into cubes
- 1 cup plain Greek yogurt
- 2 tablespoons olive oil
- 3 cloves garlic, minced
- 1 teaspoon dried oregano
- 1 teaspoon dried thyme
- 1 teaspoon ground cumin
- 1 teaspoon smoked paprika
- 1 teaspoon lemon zest
- Salt and black pepper to taste
- Wooden skewers, soaked in water

For Tzatziki:

- 1 cup Greek yogurt
- 1 cucumber, finely diced
- 2 cloves garlic, minced
- 1 tablespoon fresh dill, chopped
- 1 tablespoon extra virgin olive oil
- 1 teaspoon lemon juice
- Salt and black pepper to taste

Instructions:

1. In a bowl, mix together plain Greek yogurt, olive oil, minced garlic, dried oregano, dried thyme, ground cumin, smoked paprika, lemon zest, salt, and black pepper.
2. Add chicken cubes to the marinade, ensuring they are well-coated. Marinate in the refrigerator for at least 2 hours or overnight.
3. In another bowl, combine Greek yogurt, finely diced cucumber, minced garlic, chopped fresh dill, extra virgin olive oil, lemon juice, salt, and black pepper. Mix well.
4. Preheat the grill or grill pan over medium-high heat.
5. Thread marinated chicken cubes onto soaked wooden skewers.
6. Grill the chicken kabobs for about 6-8 minutes per side or until fully cooked.
7. Serve the Greek yogurt marinated chicken kabobs with a side of tzatziki.
8. Garnish with additional fresh dill if desired.
9. Allow to cool before storing chicken kabobs and tzatziki in meal prep containers.

Nutritional Information (per serving):

- **Carbs:** 10g
- **Sodium:** 200mg
- **Fats:** 12g
- **Protein:** 30g

Chapter 6: Vibrant Veggie Delights

Roasted Turmeric Cauliflower Steaks

Prep Time: 15 minutes | **Cook Time:** 25 minutes | **Servings:** 4

Ingredients:

- 1 large head of cauliflower
- 2 tablespoons olive oil
- 1 teaspoon ground turmeric
- 1 teaspoon ground cumin
- 1 teaspoon garlic powder
- 1 teaspoon paprika
- Salt and pepper, to taste
- Fresh parsley, for garnish

Nutritional Information (per serving):

- **Carbs:** 10g
- **Sodium:** 150mg
- **Fats:** 7g
- **Protein:** 3g

Instructions:

1. Preheat the oven to 425°F (220°C).

2. Trim the leaves and stem from the cauliflower, leaving the core intact. Place the cauliflower head on a cutting board, stem side down, and slice it into 4 steaks of even thickness.

3. In a small bowl, mix together olive oil, turmeric, cumin, garlic powder, paprika, salt, and pepper.

4. Brush both sides of each cauliflower steak with the turmeric mixture, ensuring they are well-coated.

5. Place the cauliflower steaks on a baking sheet lined with parchment paper.

6. Roast in the preheated oven for 20-25 minutes or until the edges are golden brown, flipping the steaks halfway through the cooking time.

7. Garnish with fresh parsley before serving.

Sweet Potato and Chickpea Coconut Curry

Prep Time: 20 minutes | **Cook Time:** 30 minutes | **Servings:** 6

Ingredients:

- 2 large sweet potatoes, peeled and diced
- 1 can (15 oz) chickpeas, drained and rinsed
- 1 can (14 oz) coconut milk
- 1 cup vegetable broth
- 1 onion, finely chopped
- 3 cloves garlic, minced
- 1 tablespoon fresh ginger, grated
- 1 tablespoon curry powder
- 1 teaspoon ground turmeric
- 1 teaspoon ground cumin
- 1 teaspoon coriander
- 1/2 teaspoon cinnamon
- 1 tablespoon olive oil
- Salt and pepper, to taste
- Fresh cilantro, for garnish

Nutritional Information (per serving):

- **Carbs:** 40g
- **Sodium:** 250mg
- **Fats:** 10g
- **Protein:** 7g

Instructions:

1. In a large pot, heat olive oil over medium heat. Add chopped onion, garlic, and grated ginger. Sauté until the onion is translucent.

2. Add curry powder, turmeric, cumin, coriander, and cinnamon to the pot. Stir well to coat the onion mixture with the spices.

3. Add diced sweet potatoes to the pot and cook for 5 minutes, allowing the sweet potatoes to absorb the flavors.

4. Pour in coconut milk and vegetable broth. Stir to combine, then bring the mixture to a gentle boil.

5. Reduce the heat to low and add chickpeas to the pot. Simmer for 15-20 minutes or until the sweet potatoes are tender.

6. Season with salt and pepper to taste.

7. Serve the curry over brown rice or quinoa, garnished with fresh cilantro.

<u>Grilled Eggplant and Tomato Caprese Salad</u>

Prep Time: 15 minutes | **Cook Time:** 10 minutes | **Servings:** 4

Ingredients:

- 1 large eggplant, sliced
- 4 large tomatoes, sliced
- 1/2 cup fresh basil leaves
- 1/2 cup fresh mozzarella, sliced
- 2 tablespoons balsamic glaze

- 2 tablespoons extra-virgin olive oil
- 1 clove garlic, minced
- Salt and pepper, to taste
- Pine nuts, toasted, for garnish (optional)

Nutritional Information (per serving):

- **Carbs:** 15g
- **Sodium:** 80mg

- **Fats:** 12g
- **Protein:** 6g

Instructions:

1. Preheat the grill to medium-high heat.
2. Brush both sides of the eggplant slices with olive oil and season with salt and pepper.
3. Grill the eggplant slices for 4-5 minutes on each side or until they have grill marks and are tender.
4. In a small bowl, whisk together minced garlic, balsamic glaze, and a pinch of salt.
5. On a serving platter, layer the grilled eggplant slices, tomato slices, fresh mozzarella, and basil leaves.
6. Drizzle the balsamic glaze mixture over the salad.
7. Garnish with toasted pine nuts if desired.
8. Serve immediately or store in airtight containers in the refrigerator.

<u>Rainbow Carrot and Ginger Soup</u>

Prep Time: 15 minutes | **Cook Time:** 30 minutes | **Servings:** 6

Ingredients:

- 2 lbs rainbow carrots, peeled and sliced
- 1 large onion, chopped
- 2 inches fresh ginger, peeled and sliced
- 4 cups low-sodium vegetable broth
- 1 can (14 oz) coconut milk
- 2 tablespoons olive oil
- 1 teaspoon ground turmeric
- 1/2 teaspoon ground coriander
- Salt and pepper, to taste
- Fresh cilantro, for garnish

Nutritional Information (per serving):

- **Carbs:** 18g
- **Sodium:** 180mg
- **Fats:** 10g
- **Protein:** 2g

Instructions:

1. In a large pot, heat olive oil over medium heat. Add chopped onion and sliced ginger. Sauté until the onion is soft and translucent.

2. Add sliced rainbow carrots to the pot and cook for 5 minutes, allowing the carrots to absorb the flavors.

3. Pour in low-sodium vegetable broth, coconut milk, ground turmeric, and ground coriander. Stir well to combine.

4. Bring the mixture to a boil, then reduce the heat to low and let it simmer for 20-25 minutes or until the carrots are tender.

5. Using an immersion blender, blend the soup until smooth and creamy. Alternatively, transfer the soup to a blender in batches, blending until smooth.

6. Season with salt and pepper to taste.

7. Garnish with fresh cilantro before serving.

Zucchini and Spinach Egg Muffins

Prep Time: 15 minutes | **Cook Time:** 25 minutes | **Servings:** 12

Ingredients:

- 8 large eggs
- 1 cup zucchini, grated
- 1 cup baby spinach, finely chopped
- 1/2 cup red bell pepper, finely diced
- 1/4 cup feta cheese, crumbled
- 1 teaspoon olive oil
- 1 teaspoon dried oregano
- 1/2 teaspoon garlic powder
- Salt and pepper, to taste
- Cooking spray

Nutritional Information (per serving - 1 muffin):

- **Carbs:** 2g
- **Sodium:** 120mg
- **Fats:** 8g
- **Protein:** 6g

Instructions:

1. Preheat the oven to 375°F (190°C). Grease a muffin tin with cooking spray.

2. In a skillet, heat olive oil over medium heat. Add grated zucchini and cook for 3-4 minutes until softened. Remove excess water by pressing the grated zucchini between paper towels.

3. In a large bowl, whisk the eggs. Add grated zucchini, chopped spinach, diced red bell pepper, crumbled feta cheese, dried oregano, garlic powder, salt, and pepper. Mix until well combined.

4. Spoon the egg mixture into each muffin cup, filling them nearly to the top.

5. Bake in the preheated oven for 20-25 minutes or until the tops are set and lightly golden.

6. Allow the muffins to cool for a few minutes before using a knife to loosen the edges and remove them from the tin.

7. Serve immediately or store in airtight containers in the refrigerator.

Spaghetti Squash Primavera with Basil Pesto

Prep Time: 15 minutes | **Cook Time:** 40 minutes | **Servings:** 4

Ingredients:

- 1 large spaghetti squash
- 2 cups cherry tomatoes, halved
- 1 cup bell peppers (mix of colors), sliced
- 1 cup broccoli florets
- 1/2 cup black olives, sliced
- 1/4 cup pine nuts, toasted
- 1/4 cup fresh basil leaves, chopped
- 2 tablespoons extra-virgin olive oil
- 2 cloves garlic, minced
- Salt and pepper, to taste

Nutritional Information (per serving):

- **Carbs:** 20g
- **Sodium:** 120mg
- **Fats:** 10g
- **Protein:** 4g

Instructions:

1. Preheat the oven to 375°F (190°C).

2. Cut the spaghetti squash in half lengthwise. Scoop out the seeds and pulp. Place the squash halves, cut side down, on a baking sheet. Roast in the preheated oven for 30-40 minutes or until the squash is tender and can be easily shredded with a fork.

3. While the squash is roasting, heat olive oil in a skillet over medium heat. Add minced garlic and sauté until fragrant.

4. Add bell peppers and broccoli to the skillet. Cook for 5-7 minutes or until the vegetables are tender-crisp.

5. Stir in cherry tomatoes and sliced black olives. Cook for an additional 3-4 minutes.

6. Once the spaghetti squash is done, use a fork to shred the flesh into strands.

7. Add the shredded spaghetti squash to the skillet with the sautéed vegetables. Toss everything together until well combined.

8. Season with salt and pepper to taste.

9. In a small pan, toast pine nuts over medium heat until golden brown.

10. Serve the spaghetti squash primavera topped with toasted pine nuts and chopped fresh basil.

Avocado and Tomato Cucumber Rolls

Prep Time: 20 minutes | **Cook Time:** 0 minutes | **Servings:** 4

Ingredients:

- 2 large cucumbers
- 2 avocados, sliced
- 1 cup cherry tomatoes, diced
- 1/2 red onion, finely chopped
- 1/4 cup fresh cilantro, chopped
- Juice of 1 lime
- Salt and pepper, to taste
- Sesame seeds, for garnish (optional)

Nutritional Information (per serving):

- **Carbs:** 15g
- **Sodium:** 10mg
- **Fats:** 15g
- **Protein:** 3g

Instructions:

1. Peel the cucumbers and slice them lengthwise into thin strips using a vegetable peeler or a mandoline.
2. In a bowl, combine diced cherry tomatoes, finely chopped red onion, and fresh cilantro.
3. Lay out the cucumber strips and place a slice of avocado on each strip.
4. Spoon the tomato-onion-cilantro mixture onto the avocado slices.
5. Squeeze lime juice over the rolls and sprinkle with salt and pepper.
6. Carefully roll up each cucumber strip, creating a small roll. Secure with a toothpick if needed.
7. Garnish with sesame seeds if desired.
8. Serve immediately or store in airtight containers in the refrigerator.

Roasted Beet and Goat Cheese Salad

Prep Time: 15 minutes | **Cook Time:** 45 minutes | **Servings:** 4

Ingredients:

- 4 medium-sized beets, peeled and sliced
- 6 cups mixed salad greens
- 1/2 cup goat cheese, crumbled
- 1/4 cup walnuts, chopped and toasted
- 2 tablespoons balsamic vinegar
- 2 tablespoons extra-virgin olive oil
- 1 tablespoon honey
- Salt and pepper, to taste
- Fresh thyme leaves, for garnish

Nutritional Information (per serving):

- **Carbs:** 20g
- **Sodium:** 150mg
- **Fats:** 10g
- **Protein:** 5g

Instructions:

1. Preheat the oven to 400°F (200°C).
2. Peel and slice the beets into uniform pieces.
3. Place the sliced beets on a baking sheet, drizzle with olive oil, and season with salt and pepper. Toss to coat evenly.
4. Roast the beets in the preheated oven for 40-45 minutes or until they are tender. Toss them halfway through the cooking time.
5. While the beets are roasting, prepare the salad. In a large bowl, combine mixed salad greens, crumbled goat cheese, and chopped toasted walnuts.
6. In a small bowl, whisk together balsamic vinegar, olive oil, and honey to create the dressing.
7. Once the beets are done, let them cool slightly before adding them to the salad.
8. Drizzle the balsamic vinaigrette over the salad and gently toss to combine.
9. Garnish with fresh thyme leaves.
10. Serve immediately or store in airtight containers in the refrigerator.

Brussels Sprouts and Almond Stir-Fry

Prep Time: 15 minutes | **Cook Time:** 15 minutes | **Servings:** 4

Ingredients:

- 1 lb Brussels sprouts, trimmed and halved
- 1 cup almonds, sliced and toasted
- 1 red bell pepper, thinly sliced
- 1 yellow bell pepper, thinly sliced
- 2 tablespoons olive oil
- 3 cloves garlic, minced
- 1 tablespoon fresh ginger, grated
- 2 tablespoons low-sodium soy sauce
- 1 tablespoon rice vinegar
- 1 teaspoon honey
- Salt and pepper, to taste
- Sesame seeds, for garnish (optional)
- Green onions, sliced, for garnish (optional)

Nutritional Information (per serving):

- **Carbs:** 18g
- **Sodium:** 180mg
- **Fats:** 15g
- **Protein:** 9g

Instructions:

1. Trim the Brussels sprouts and cut them in half.

2. In a large skillet or wok, heat olive oil over medium-high heat.

3. Add minced garlic and grated ginger to the skillet. Sauté until fragrant.

4. Add Brussels sprouts, red bell pepper, and yellow bell pepper to the skillet. Stir-fry for about 8-10 minutes until the Brussels sprouts are tender-crisp.

5. In a small bowl, whisk together low-sodium soy sauce, rice vinegar, and honey.

6. Pour the sauce over the stir-fry and toss to coat the vegetables evenly.

7. Season with salt and pepper to taste.

8. Toast the sliced almonds in a dry pan until golden brown, then sprinkle them over the stir-fry.

9. Garnish with sesame seeds and sliced green onions if desired.

10. Serve immediately or store in airtight containers in the refrigerator.

Cabbage and Cashew Coleslaw with Turmeric Dressing

Prep Time: 20 minutes | **Cook Time:** 0 minutes | **Servings:** 6

Ingredients:

- 1 small head green cabbage, shredded
- 2 carrots, julienned
- 1 cup raw cashews, chopped and toasted
- 1/2 cup fresh cilantro, chopped
- 1/4 cup red onion, thinly sliced
- 1/4 cup apple cider vinegar
- 2 tablespoons extra-virgin olive oil
- 1 tablespoon raw honey
- 1 teaspoon ground turmeric
- Salt and pepper, to taste
- Sesame seeds, for garnish (optional)

Nutritional Information (per serving):

- **Carbs:** 18g
- **Sodium:** 80mg
- **Fats:** 12g
- **Protein:** 5g

Instructions:

1. In a large mixing bowl, combine shredded green cabbage, julienned carrots, chopped and toasted cashews, chopped cilantro, and thinly sliced red onion.

2. In a small bowl, whisk together apple cider vinegar, extra-virgin olive oil, raw honey, ground turmeric, salt, and pepper to create the dressing.

3. Pour the turmeric dressing over the cabbage mixture.

4. Toss the ingredients until the coleslaw is evenly coated with the dressing.

5. Adjust salt and pepper to taste.

6. Garnish with sesame seeds if desired.

7. Serve immediately or store in airtight containers in the refrigerator.

<u>Roasted Red Pepper and Lentil Patties</u>

Prep Time: 30 minutes | **Cook Time:** 25 minutes | **Servings:** 4

Ingredients:

- 1 cup dry red lentils, rinsed and drained
- 2 cups vegetable broth
- 2 large red bell peppers, roasted and finely diced
- 1 cup rolled oats, pulsed into a coarse powder
- 1/2 cup red onion, finely chopped
- 2 cloves garlic, minced
- 2 teaspoons ground cumin
- 1 teaspoon ground coriander
- 1/2 teaspoon smoked paprika
- Salt and pepper, to taste
- 2 tablespoons olive oil, for cooking

Nutritional Information (per serving - 2 patties):

- **Carbs:** 30g
- **Sodium:** 180mg
- **Fats:** 7g
- **Protein:** 13g

Instructions:

1. In a medium saucepan, combine red lentils and vegetable broth. Bring to a boil, then reduce heat and simmer for 15-20 minutes or until lentils are tender and most of the liquid is absorbed.

2. While lentils are cooking, roast the red bell peppers. Once roasted, finely dice them.

3. In a large mixing bowl, combine cooked red lentils, diced roasted red peppers, coarse oat powder, finely chopped red onion, minced garlic, ground cumin, ground coriander, smoked paprika, salt, and pepper.

4. Mix the ingredients until well combined. Let the mixture sit for 10 minutes to absorb flavors.

5. Form the mixture into patties. If the mixture is too wet, add a bit more oat powder.

6. In a skillet, heat olive oil over medium heat.

7. Cook the lentil patties for 4-5 minutes per side or until golden brown and cooked through.

8. Serve immediately or let them cool before storing in airtight containers in the refrigerator.

Artichoke and Spinach Stuffed Mushrooms

Prep Time: 20 minutes | **Cook Time:** 25 minutes | **Servings:** 4

Ingredients:

- 20 large mushrooms, stems removed and reserved
- 1 cup frozen chopped spinach, thawed and drained
- 1 can (14 oz) artichoke hearts, drained and finely chopped
- 1/2 cup grated Parmesan cheese
- 1/2 cup plain Greek yogurt
- 2 cloves garlic, minced
- 2 tablespoons extra-virgin olive oil
- 1 teaspoon dried oregano
- Salt and pepper, to taste
- Fresh parsley, chopped, for garnish

Nutritional Information (per serving - 5 mushrooms):

- **Carbs:** 10g
- **Sodium:** 150mg
- **Fats:** 8g
- **Protein:** 6g

Instructions:

1. Preheat the oven to 375°F (190°C). Grease a baking dish with olive oil.
2. Clean the mushrooms and remove the stems. Finely chop the mushroom stems.
3. In a skillet, heat olive oil over medium heat. Add minced garlic and chopped mushroom stems. Sauté until the mushrooms release their moisture.
4. Add thawed and drained chopped spinach to the skillet. Cook until any excess moisture evaporates.
5. In a bowl, combine the sautéed mixture with finely chopped artichoke hearts, grated Parmesan cheese, plain Greek yogurt, dried oregano, salt, and pepper.
6. Mix well until all ingredients are evenly incorporated.
7. Stuff each mushroom cap with the spinach and artichoke mixture.
8. Place the stuffed mushrooms in the prepared baking dish.
9. Bake in the preheated oven for 20-25 minutes or until the mushrooms are tender and the filling is golden brown.
10. Garnish with chopped fresh parsley before serving.

Lemon-Garlic Roasted Broccoli and Cauliflower

Prep Time: 15 minutes | **Cook Time:** 20 minutes | **Servings:** 4

Ingredients:

- 1 lb broccoli florets
- 1 lb cauliflower florets
- 3 cloves garlic, minced
- Zest of 1 lemon
- Juice of 1 lemon
- 3 tablespoons extra-virgin olive oil
- 1 teaspoon dried thyme
- Salt and pepper, to taste
- Lemon slices, for garnish (optional)

Nutritional Information (per serving):

- **Carbs:** 15g
- **Sodium:** 80mg
- **Fats:** 8g
- **Protein:** 5g

Instructions:

1. Preheat the oven to 425°F (220°C). Line a baking sheet with parchment paper.
2. In a large bowl, combine broccoli florets and cauliflower florets.
3. In a small bowl, whisk together minced garlic, lemon zest, lemon juice, extra-virgin olive oil, dried thyme, salt, and pepper to create the marinade.
4. Pour the marinade over the broccoli and cauliflower, ensuring even coating.
5. Spread the vegetables in a single layer on the prepared baking sheet.
6. Roast in the preheated oven for 20 minutes or until the edges are golden brown and the vegetables are tender. Toss halfway through for even roasting.
7. Garnish with lemon slices if desired.
8. Serve immediately or store in airtight containers in the refrigerator.

Asparagus and Sun-Dried Tomato Frittata

Prep Time: 15 minutes | **Cook Time:** 25 minutes | **Servings:** 6

Ingredients:

- 8 large eggs
- 1 bunch asparagus, trimmed and cut into 1-inch pieces
- 1/2 cup sun-dried tomatoes, drained and chopped
- 1/2 cup feta cheese, crumbled

- 1/4 cup fresh basil, chopped
- 1/4 cup red onion, finely chopped
- 2 cloves garlic, minced
- 2 tablespoons extra-virgin olive oil
- 1 teaspoon dried oregano
- Salt and pepper, to taste

Nutritional Information (per serving):

- **Carbs:** 5g
- **Sodium:** 180mg

- **Fats:** 12g
- **Protein:** 12g

Instructions:

1. Preheat the oven to 375°F (190°C).

2. In a skillet, heat olive oil over medium heat. Add minced garlic and chopped red onion. Sauté until softened.

3. Add asparagus pieces to the skillet and cook for 3-4 minutes until they are slightly tender.

4. In a bowl, whisk together eggs, dried oregano, salt, and pepper.

5. Pour the egg mixture over the asparagus in the skillet.

6. Sprinkle chopped sun-dried tomatoes, crumbled feta cheese, and chopped fresh basil evenly over the eggs.

7. Cook on the stovetop for 3-4 minutes until the edges set.

8. Transfer the skillet to the preheated oven and bake for 18-20 minutes or until the frittata is set in the middle.

9. Once cooked, let it cool before slicing.

10. Serve immediately or store in airtight containers in the refrigerator.

<u>Sauteed Kale and Walnut Pesto Pasta</u>

Prep Time: 15 minutes | **Cook Time:** 20 minutes | **Servings:** 4

Ingredients:

- 8 oz whole wheat pasta
- 4 cups kale, stems removed and leaves chopped
- 1 cup walnuts, toasted
- 1/2 cup Parmesan cheese, grated
- 2 cloves garlic, minced
-)

- 1/2 cup extra-virgin olive oil
- Juice of 1 lemon
- Salt and pepper, to taste
- Red pepper flakes, for garnish (optional

Nutritional Information (per serving):

- **Carbs:** 45g
- **Sodium:** 120mg
- **Fats:** 28g
- **Protein:** 12g

Instructions:

1. Cook the whole wheat pasta according to package instructions. Drain and set aside.

2. In a skillet, heat olive oil over medium heat. Add minced garlic and sauté until fragrant.

3. Add chopped kale to the skillet. Saute for 5-7 minutes until the kale is wilted and tender.

4. In a food processor, combine toasted walnuts, grated Parmesan cheese, and sautéed kale. Pulse until coarsely chopped.

5. With the food processor running, stream in the extra-virgin olive oil until the pesto reaches your desired consistency.

6. Add lemon juice, salt, and pepper to the pesto. Pulse to combine.

7. Toss the cooked pasta with the kale and walnut pesto until well coated.

8. Garnish with red pepper flakes if desired.

9. Serve immediately or store in airtight containers in the refrigerator.

Miso-Glazed Japanese Eggplant

Prep Time: 15 minutes | **Cook Time:** 20 minutes | **Servings:** 4

Ingredients:

- 4 Japanese eggplants, halved lengthwise
- 1/4 cup white miso paste
- 2 tablespoons mirin
- 2 tablespoons rice vinegar
- 1 tablespoon maple syrup
- 2 teaspoons sesame oil
- 1 tablespoon sesame seeds, toasted
- Green onions, sliced, for garnish
- Fresh cilantro, chopped, for garnish (optional)

Nutritional Information (per serving):

- **Carbs:** 15g
- **Sodium:** 200mg
- **Fats:** 5g
- **Protein:** 2g

Instructions:

1. Preheat the oven to 400°F (200°C).
2. Score the flesh of the halved Japanese eggplants with a crosshatch pattern.
3. In a bowl, whisk together white miso paste, mirin, rice vinegar, maple syrup, and sesame oil to create the glaze.
4. Place the eggplants on a baking sheet and generously brush them with the miso glaze, ensuring it gets into the scores.
5. Roast in the preheated oven for 15-20 minutes or until the eggplants are tender and the tops are golden brown.
6. While the eggplants are roasting, toast sesame seeds in a dry pan until they become fragrant.
7. Once out of the oven, sprinkle the miso-glazed eggplants with toasted sesame seeds.
8. Garnish with sliced green onions and chopped cilantro if desired.
9. Serve immediately or store in airtight containers in the refrigerator.

Ratatouille with Herbed Quinoa

Prep Time: 20 minutes | **Cook Time:** 40 minutes | **Servings:** 6

Ingredients:

For Ratatouille:

- 1 large eggplant, diced
- 2 zucchini, sliced
- 2 yellow squash, sliced
- 1 large red bell pepper, diced
- 1 large yellow bell pepper, diced
- 1 red onion, diced
- 4 cloves garlic, minced
- 1 can (28 oz) crushed tomatoes
- 2 tablespoons tomato paste
- 2 teaspoons dried oregano
- 2 teaspoons dried thyme
- 1 teaspoon dried rosemary
- 1 teaspoon dried basil
- Salt and pepper, to taste
- 2 tablespoons olive oil

For Herbed Quinoa:

- 1 cup quinoa, rinsed
- 2 cups vegetable broth
- 1 teaspoon dried thyme
- 1 teaspoon dried rosemary
- Salt and pepper, to taste

Nutritional Information (per serving):

- **Carbs:** 40g
- **Sodium:** 280mg
- **Fats:** 8g
- **Protein:** 6g

Instructions:

1. Preheat the oven to 375°F (190°C).

2. In a large baking dish, combine diced eggplant, sliced zucchini, sliced yellow squash, diced red bell pepper, diced yellow bell pepper, diced red onion, and minced garlic.

3. In a bowl, mix crushed tomatoes, tomato paste, dried oregano, dried thyme, dried rosemary, dried basil, salt, and pepper.

4. Pour the tomato mixture over the vegetables in the baking dish. Toss to coat evenly.

5. Drizzle olive oil over the top and toss again to ensure all vegetables are coated.

6. Roast in the preheated oven for 35-40 minutes or until the vegetables are tender, stirring halfway through.

7. In a saucepan, combine rinsed quinoa, vegetable broth, dried thyme, dried rosemary, salt, and pepper.

8. Bring to a boil, then reduce heat, cover, and simmer for 15-20 minutes or until quinoa is cooked and liquid is absorbed.

9. Fluff the quinoa with a fork.

10. Spoon a portion of herbed quinoa onto a plate.

11. Top with a generous serving of ratatouille.

12. Garnish with fresh herbs if desired.

Chapter 7: Healthy Fats Feast

Avocado and Black Bean Lettuce Wraps

Prep Time: 15 minutes | Cook Time: 10 minutes | Servings: 4

Ingredients:

- 1 cup dried black beans, soaked overnight and cooked
- 2 ripe avocados, diced
- 1 cup cherry tomatoes, halved
- 1/2 red onion, finely chopped
- 1 cup corn kernels, cooked
- 1/4 cup fresh cilantro, chopped
- 2 cloves garlic, minced
- Juice of 2 limes
- 1 teaspoon ground cumin
- Salt and pepper to taste
- 8 large lettuce leaves (such as iceberg or butter lettuce)

Instructions:

1. In a large mixing bowl, combine the cooked black beans, diced avocados, cherry tomatoes, finely chopped red onion, cooked corn kernels, chopped cilantro, minced garlic, lime juice, ground cumin, salt, and pepper. Toss gently to mix well.

2. Lay out the large lettuce leaves on a clean surface. Spoon the avocado and black bean mixture evenly onto each lettuce leaf.

3. Fold the sides of the lettuce leaves over the filling and then roll them up tightly, creating a wrap.

4. Secure each wrap with toothpicks if needed.

5. Store the wraps in airtight containers, placing parchment paper between layers to prevent sticking. Refrigerate for up to 3 days.

Nutritional Information (per serving):

- Carbs: 30g
- Sodium: 180mg
- Fats: 15g
- Protein: 8g

Smoked Salmon and Avocado Sushi Rolls

Prep Time: 20 minutes | Cook Time: 0 minutes (no cooking required) | Servings: 4

Ingredients:

- 2 cups sushi rice, cooked and seasoned with rice vinegar
- 4 nori (seaweed) sheets
- 8 ounces smoked salmon, thinly sliced
- 2 ripe avocados, sliced
- 1 cucumber, julienned
- 1/4 cup pickled ginger
- 1/4 cup reduced-sodium soy sauce
- 1 tablespoon sesame seeds
- Wasabi and soy sauce for serving (optional)

Instructions:

1. Lay a bamboo sushi rolling mat on a flat surface. Place a sheet of plastic wrap on the mat.

2. Put one nori sheet, shiny side down, onto the plastic wrap.

3. Moisten your hands with water to prevent sticking, then evenly spread a layer of sushi rice over the nori, leaving a small border at the top.

4. Arrange slices of smoked salmon, avocado, and julienned cucumber horizontally on the rice.

5. Using the bamboo mat, roll the sushi tightly from the bottom, using the plastic wrap to help shape and compress the roll.

6. Seal the edge with a bit of water.

7. Repeat the process for the remaining nori sheets.

8. With a sharp knife moistened with water, slice each roll into bite-sized pieces.

9. Serve the smoked salmon and avocado sushi rolls with pickled ginger, reduced-sodium soy sauce, sesame seeds, and, if desired, wasabi.

10. Store the sushi rolls in airtight containers in the refrigerator for up to 2 days.

Nutritional Information (per serving):

- Carbs: 40g
- Sodium: 300mg
- Fats: 10g
- Protein: 15g

<u>Almond-Crusted Halibut with Mango Salsa</u>

Prep Time: 15 minutes | Cook Time: 15 minutes | Servings: 4

Ingredients:

For the Almond-Crusted Halibut:

- 4 halibut fillets
- 1 cup almond flour
- 1/2 cup almonds, finely chopped

For the Mango Salsa:

- 2 ripe mangoes, diced
- 1 red bell pepper, diced
- 1/4 red onion, finely chopped

- 1 teaspoon paprika
- 1/2 teaspoon garlic powder
- Salt and pepper to taste
- 2 eggs, beaten
- 1/4 cup fresh cilantro, chopped
- Juice of 1 lime
- Salt to taste

Instructions:

Almond-Crusted Halibut:

1. Preheat the oven to 400°F (200°C). Line a baking sheet with parchment paper.
2. In a shallow bowl, combine almond flour, finely chopped almonds, paprika, garlic powder, salt, and pepper.
3. Dip each halibut fillet into the beaten eggs, ensuring an even coating.
4. Press the egg-coated fillets into the almond mixture, coating both sides thoroughly.
5. Place the coated fillets on the prepared baking sheet and bake for 15 minutes or until the crust is golden brown and the fish flakes easily with a fork.

Mango Salsa:

1. In a bowl, combine diced mangoes, diced red bell pepper, finely chopped red onion, chopped cilantro, lime juice, and salt. Mix well.
2. Refrigerate the mango salsa until ready to serve.

Serving:

1. Plate the almond-crusted halibut fillets and top each with a generous spoonful of mango salsa.
2. Garnish with additional cilantro if desired.

Nutritional Information (per serving):

- Carbs: 20g
- Sodium: 300mg

- Fats: 15g
- Protein: 30g

Chia Seed Pudding Parfait with Berries

Prep Time: 10 minutes (+overnight chilling) | Cook Time: 0 minutes | Servings: 4

Ingredients:

For the Chia Seed Pudding:

- 1/2 cup chia seeds
- 2 cups unsweetened almond milk
- 1 teaspoon vanilla extract
- 1 tablespoon maple syrup

For the Parfait:

- 2 cups mixed berries (strawberries, blueberries, raspberries)
- 1 cup Greek yogurt (unsweetened)
- 1/4 cup almonds, sliced
- 1 tablespoon honey (optional)

Instructions:

Chia Seed Pudding:

1. In a bowl, whisk together chia seeds, unsweetened almond milk, maple syrup, and vanilla extract.
2. Cover the bowl and refrigerate overnight or for at least 4 hours to allow the chia seeds to absorb the liquid and form a pudding-like consistency.

Parfait Assembly:

1. In serving glasses or jars, layer the chia seed pudding with Greek yogurt.
2. Top the layers with mixed berries and sliced almonds.
3. Drizzle honey on top if desired.
4. Repeat the layering process until the glasses are filled, finishing with a layer of berries and a sprinkle of sliced almonds.
5. Refrigerate until ready to serve or store in airtight containers for meal prep.

Nutritional Information (per serving):

- Carbs: 30g
- Sodium: 50mg
- Fats: 15g
- Protein: 10g

<u>Walnut-Crusted Chicken Salad with Raspberry Vinaigrette</u>

Prep Time: 20 minutes | Cook Time: 15 minutes | Servings: 4

Ingredients:

For the Walnut-Crusted Chicken:

- 4 boneless, skinless chicken breasts
- 1 cup walnuts, finely chopped
- 1/2 cup whole wheat breadcrumbs
- 1 teaspoon dried thyme
- 1/2 teaspoon garlic powder
- Salt and pepper to taste
- 2 eggs, beaten
- Olive oil for cooking

For the Raspberry Vinaigrette:

- 1/2 cup fresh raspberries
- 3 tablespoons olive oil
- 2 tablespoons balsamic vinegar
- 1 tablespoon honey
- 1 teaspoon Dijon mustard
- Salt and pepper to taste

For the Salad:

- 8 cups mixed salad greens
- 1 cup cherry tomatoes, halved
- 1 cucumber, sliced
- 1/2 red onion, thinly sliced
- 1/2 cup feta cheese, crumbled (optional)

Instructions:

1. Preheat the oven to 375°F (190°C).
2. In a bowl, combine finely chopped walnuts, whole wheat breadcrumbs, dried thyme, garlic powder, salt, and pepper.
3. Dip each chicken breast into the beaten eggs, coating both sides.
4. Press the egg-coated chicken breasts into the walnut mixture, ensuring an even coating.
5. In a skillet, heat olive oil over medium heat. Cook the chicken breasts for 3-4 minutes on each side until golden brown.
6. Transfer the browned chicken breasts to a baking sheet and bake in the preheated oven for about 10 minutes or until the internal temperature reaches 165°F (74°C).
7. In a blender, combine fresh raspberries, olive oil, balsamic vinegar, honey, Dijon mustard, salt, and pepper. Blend until smooth.
8. Strain the vinaigrette through a fine mesh sieve to remove seeds.
9. In a large bowl, toss the mixed salad greens, cherry tomatoes, sliced cucumber, and thinly sliced red onion.
10. Slice the walnut-crusted chicken and place it on top of the salad.
11. Drizzle the raspberry vinaigrette over the salad and chicken.
12. Optionally, sprinkle crumbled feta cheese on top.

Nutritional Information (per serving):

- Carbs: 25g
- Sodium: 250mg
- Fats: 20g
- Protein: 30g

Pistachio-Crusted Cod with Lemon-Dill Aioli

Prep Time: 15 minutes | Cook Time: 12 minutes | Servings: 4

Ingredients:

For the Pistachio-Crusted Cod:

- 4 cod fillets
- 1 cup pistachios, finely chopped
- 1/2 cup whole wheat breadcrumbs
- 1 teaspoon dried thyme
- 1/2 teaspoon garlic powder
- Salt and pepper to taste
- 2 eggs, beaten
- Olive oil for cooking

For the Lemon-Dill Aioli:

- 1/2 cup plain Greek yogurt (unsweetened)
- 1 tablespoon fresh dill, finely chopped
- 1 teaspoon lemon zest
- 1 tablespoon lemon juice
- 1 clove garlic, minced
- Salt and pepper to taste

Instructions:

Pistachio-Crusted Cod:

1. Preheat the oven to 375°F (190°C).

2. In a bowl, combine finely chopped pistachios, whole wheat breadcrumbs, dried thyme, garlic powder, salt, and pepper.

3. Dip each cod fillet into the beaten eggs, coating both sides.

4. Press the egg-coated cod fillets into the pistachio mixture, ensuring an even coating.

5. In an oven-safe skillet, heat olive oil over medium heat. Cook the cod fillets for 2-3 minutes on each side until golden brown.

6. Transfer the skillet to the preheated oven and bake for an additional 8-10 minutes or until the cod flakes easily with a fork.

7. In a small bowl, mix together plain Greek yogurt, finely chopped fresh dill, lemon zest, lemon juice, minced garlic, salt, and pepper. Set aside.

8. Plate the pistachio-crusted cod fillets.

9. Drizzle each fillet with the lemon-dill aioli.

Nutritional Information (per serving):

- Carbs: 15g
- Sodium: 200mg
- Fats: 15g
- Protein: 30g

Avocado and Chickpea Stuffed Bell Peppers

Prep Time: 20 minutes | Cook Time: 25 minutes | Servings: 4

Ingredients:

- 4 bell peppers, halved and seeds removed
- 1 can (15 oz) chickpeas, drained and rinsed
- 2 avocados, diced
- 1 cup cherry tomatoes, diced
- 1/2 red onion, finely chopped
- 2 cloves garlic, minced
- 1/4 cup fresh cilantro, chopped
- 1 teaspoon cumin
- 1/2 teaspoon smoked paprika
- Salt and pepper to taste
- 2 tablespoons olive oil
- 1 cup quinoa, cooked
- 1/4 cup pine nuts, toasted (optional)

Instructions:

1. Preheat the oven to 375°F (190°C).
2. Place the bell pepper halves in a baking dish.
3. In a large bowl, combine chickpeas, diced avocados, diced cherry tomatoes, finely chopped red onion, minced garlic, chopped cilantro, cumin, smoked paprika, salt, and pepper. Mix well.
4. Spoon the chickpea and avocado mixture into each bell pepper half.
5. Drizzle olive oil over the stuffed peppers.
6. Bake in the preheated oven for 25 minutes or until the peppers are tender.
7. While the peppers are baking, prepare the quinoa according to package instructions.
8. Serve the stuffed bell peppers over a bed of cooked quinoa.
9. Optionally, sprinkle toasted pine nuts on top for added crunch.

Nutritional Information (per serving):

- Carbs: 40g
- Sodium: 150mg
- Fats: 20g
- Protein: 10g

Pomegranate Guacamole with Jicama Chips

Prep Time: 15 minutes | Cook Time: 0 minutes | Servings: 4

Ingredients:

For the Pomegranate Guacamole:

- 3 ripe avocados, diced
- 1/2 cup pomegranate seeds
- 1/4 cup red onion, finely chopped

- 1/4 cup fresh cilantro, chopped
- 1 jalapeño, seeds removed and finely chopped
- Juice of 2 limes
- Salt and pepper to taste

For the Jicama Chips:

- 1 medium jicama, peeled and sliced into thin rounds
- 1 tablespoon olive oil

- 1 teaspoon smoked paprika
- 1/2 teaspoon cumin
- Salt to taste

Instructions:

Pomegranate Guacamole:

1. In a bowl, combine diced avocados, pomegranate seeds, finely chopped red onion, chopped cilantro, chopped jalapeño, lime juice, salt, and pepper. Mix gently.

2. Adjust salt and pepper according to taste.

Jicama Chips:

1. In a large bowl, toss jicama rounds with olive oil, smoked paprika, cumin, and salt.

2. Arrange the seasoned jicama rounds on a serving platter.

3. Optionally, chill the guacamole and jicama chips in the refrigerator for about 30 minutes before serving.

Serving:

1. Serve the pomegranate guacamole in a bowl alongside the jicama chips.

2. Use the jicama chips for scooping and enjoying the flavorful guacamole.

Nutritional Information (per serving):

- Carbs: 20g
- Sodium: 100mg
- Fats: 15g
- Protein: 3g

Salmon and Avocado Quinoa Bowl

Prep Time: 15 minutes | Cook Time: 15 minutes | Servings: 4

Ingredients:

- 1 cup quinoa, rinsed
- 4 salmon fillets
- 2 tablespoons olive oil
- 1 teaspoon smoked paprika
- 1 teaspoon garlic powder
- Salt and pepper to taste
- 2 avocados, sliced
- 1 cucumber, diced
- 1 cup cherry tomatoes, halved
- 1/4 cup red onion, finely chopped
- 1/4 cup fresh cilantro, chopped
- Juice of 2 limes

Instructions:

1. In a medium saucepan, combine rinsed quinoa with 2 cups of water. Bring to a boil, then reduce heat to low, cover, and simmer for 15 minutes or until the quinoa is cooked and water is absorbed.

2. Preheat the oven to 400°F (200°C).

3. Place the salmon fillets on a baking sheet lined with parchment paper.

4. Drizzle olive oil over the salmon fillets and sprinkle with smoked paprika, garlic powder, salt, and pepper.

5. Bake the salmon in the preheated oven for 12-15 minutes or until it flakes easily with a fork.

6. While the quinoa and salmon are cooking, prepare the vegetables. Combine sliced avocados, diced cucumber, halved cherry tomatoes, finely chopped red onion, and chopped cilantro in a bowl.

7. Once the quinoa is cooked, fluff it with a fork and divide it among four bowls.

8. Top each bowl with a baked salmon fillet and the avocado-vegetable mixture.

9. Drizzle lime juice over each bowl for added freshness.

Nutritional Information (per serving):

- Carbs: 40g
- Sodium: 150mg
- Fats: 20g
- Protein: 30g

Coconut-Curry Almond Butter Stir-Fry

Prep Time: 20 minutes | Cook Time: 15 minutes | Servings: 4

Ingredients:

- 1 cup quinoa, rinsed
- 1 pound boneless, skinless chicken breasts, thinly sliced
- 2 tablespoons coconut oil
- 1 red bell pepper, sliced
- 1 yellow bell pepper, sliced
- 1 cup snap peas, ends trimmed
- 1 carrot, julienned
- 1/2 cup unsalted almond butter
- 1 can (13.5 oz) coconut milk
- 3 tablespoons low-sodium soy sauce
- 2 tablespoons curry powder
- 1 teaspoon ginger, minced
- 2 cloves garlic, minced
- 1 tablespoon honey
- Salt and pepper to taste
- Fresh cilantro for garnish
- Sliced almonds for garnish

Instructions:

1. In a medium saucepan, combine rinsed quinoa with 2 cups of water. Bring to a boil, then reduce heat to low, cover, and simmer for 15 minutes or until the quinoa is cooked and water is absorbed.

2. In a large wok or skillet, heat coconut oil over medium-high heat.

3. Add the sliced chicken breasts to the wok and stir-fry until cooked through. Remove the cooked chicken from the wok and set aside.

4. In the same wok, add more coconut oil if needed. Stir-fry the sliced red and yellow bell peppers, snap peas, and julienned carrot until they are crisp-tender.

5. In a bowl, whisk together almond butter, coconut milk, low-sodium soy sauce, curry powder, minced ginger, minced garlic, honey, salt, and pepper.

6. Pour the almond butter mixture into the wok with the vegetables. Add the cooked chicken back into the wok. Stir to coat everything evenly and simmer for a few minutes until heated through.

7. Serve the stir-fry over a bed of cooked quinoa.

8. Garnish with fresh cilantro and sliced almonds.

Nutritional Information (per serving):

- Carbs: 45g
- Sodium: 300mg
- Fats: 25g
- Protein: 30g

Greek Salad with Kalamata Olive Hummus

Prep Time: 20 minutes | Cook Time: 0 minutes | Servings: 4

Ingredients:

For the Greek Salad:

- 1 large cucumber, diced
- 2 cups cherry tomatoes, halved
- 1 red bell pepper, diced

For the Kalamata Olive Hummus:

- 1 can (15 oz) chickpeas, drained and rinsed
- 1/4 cup Kalamata olives, pitted
- 2 tablespoons tahini

- 1/2 red onion, thinly sliced
- 1 cup Kalamata olives, pitted and sliced
- 1 cup feta cheese, crumbled
- 1/4 cup fresh parsley, chopped

- 2 cloves garlic, minced
- Juice of 1 lemon
- 3 tablespoons olive oil
- Salt and pepper to taste

Instructions:

Greek Salad:

1. In a large bowl, combine diced cucumber, halved cherry tomatoes, diced red bell pepper, thinly sliced red onion, sliced Kalamata olives, crumbled feta cheese, and chopped fresh parsley.
2. Toss the salad ingredients together until well mixed.

Kalamata Olive Hummus:

1. In a food processor, combine drained and rinsed chickpeas, Kalamata olives, tahini, minced garlic, lemon juice, olive oil, salt, and pepper.
2. Blend until smooth, scraping down the sides as needed.

Serving:

1. Plate the Greek salad in individual serving bowls.
2. Drizzle each salad with the Kalamata olive hummus.
3. Optionally, garnish with additional feta cheese and fresh parsley.

Nutritional Information (per serving):

- Carbs: 25g
- Sodium: 400mg
- Fats: 18g
- Protein: 10g

Walnut and Cranberry Stuffed Acorn Squash

Prep Time: 20 minutes | Cook Time: 40 minutes | Servings: 4

Ingredients:

- 2 acorn squashes, halved and seeds removed
- 1 cup quinoa, rinsed
- 2 cups vegetable broth
- 1 cup walnuts, chopped
- 1/2 cup dried cranberries
- 1/4 cup fresh parsley, chopped
- 1/4 cup red onion, finely chopped
- 2 tablespoons olive oil
- 1 teaspoon ground cinnamon
- 1/2 teaspoon ground nutmeg
- Salt and pepper to taste

Instructions:

1. Preheat the oven to 400°F (200°C).

2. Place the acorn squash halves, cut side down, on a baking sheet. Bake for 20-25 minutes or until the squash is fork-tender.

3. In a saucepan, combine rinsed quinoa and vegetable broth. Bring to a boil, then reduce heat to low, cover, and simmer for 15 minutes or until the quinoa is cooked and water is absorbed.

4. In a large bowl, combine cooked quinoa, chopped walnuts, dried cranberries, chopped fresh parsley, finely chopped red onion, olive oil, ground cinnamon, ground nutmeg, salt, and pepper. Mix well.

5. Once the acorn squash halves are baked, carefully flip them over.

6. Fill each acorn squash half with the quinoa mixture, pressing down lightly to pack it.

7. Return the stuffed acorn squash to the oven and bake for an additional 15 minutes or until the filling is heated through and the tops are golden.

8. Optionally, garnish with additional chopped parsley before serving.

Nutritional Information (per serving):

- Carbs: 45g
- Sodium: 300mg
- Fats: 18g
- Protein: 10g

Caprese Avocado Toast with Balsamic Glaze

Prep Time: 10 minutes | Cook Time: 5 minutes | Servings: 4

Ingredients:

- 4 slices whole-grain bread
- 2 ripe avocados, sliced
- 2 medium tomatoes, sliced
- 1 cup fresh mozzarella, sliced
- Fresh basil leaves
- Balsamic glaze
- Olive oil for drizzling
- Salt and pepper to taste

Instructions:

1. Toast the whole-grain bread slices to your liking.
2. While the bread is toasting, prepare the avocado, tomatoes, and fresh mozzarella.
3. Once the toast is ready, place avocado slices on each slice of bread, spreading them evenly.
4. Top the avocado with tomato slices, followed by slices of fresh mozzarella.
5. Place fresh basil leaves on top of the mozzarella.
6. Drizzle balsamic glaze over each toast for added flavor.
7. Finish with a light drizzle of olive oil.
8. Sprinkle salt and pepper to taste.

Nutritional Information (per serving):

- Carbs: 30g
- Sodium: 200mg
- Fats: 20g
- Protein: 12g

Cucumber and Avocado Gazpacho

Prep Time: 15 minutes (+chilling time) | Cook Time: 0 minutes | Servings: 4

Ingredients:

- 4 large cucumbers, peeled and diced
- 2 ripe avocados, peeled and diced
- 1 green bell pepper, diced
- 1/2 red onion, diced
- 2 cloves garlic, minced
- 1/4 cup fresh cilantro, chopped
- 3 cups vegetable broth (low-sodium)
- 1/4 cup olive oil
- Juice of 2 limes
- Salt and pepper to taste
- Greek yogurt for garnish (optional)
- Additional cilantro for garnish (optional)

Instructions:

1. In a large bowl, combine diced cucumbers, diced avocados, diced green bell pepper, diced red onion, minced garlic, and chopped fresh cilantro.

2. In a blender, puree half of the vegetable mixture with vegetable broth until smooth.

3. Add the remaining vegetable mixture to the blender and pulse a few times, leaving some texture.

4. Pour the blended mixture back into the large bowl.

5. Stir in olive oil and lime juice.

6. Season the gazpacho with salt and pepper to taste. Refrigerate for at least 2 hours or until well chilled.

7. Before serving, taste and adjust seasoning if needed.

8. Serve the cucumber and avocado gazpacho chilled, garnished with a dollop of Greek yogurt and additional cilantro if desired.

Nutritional Information (per serving):

- Carbs: 20g
- Sodium: 150mg
- Fats: 15g
- Protein: 4g

Almond-Crusted Chicken Caesar Salad

Prep Time: 20 minutes | Cook Time: 20 minutes | Servings: 4

Ingredients:

For the Almond-Crusted Chicken:

- 4 boneless, skinless chicken breasts
- 1 cup almond flour
- 2 teaspoons dried oregano

For the Caesar Salad:

- 2 heads romaine lettuce, chopped
- 1 cup cherry tomatoes, halved
- 1/2 cup Parmesan cheese, shaved
- 1/4 cup extra-virgin olive oil
- Juice of 1 lemon

- 1 teaspoon garlic powder
- Salt and pepper to taste
- 2 eggs, beaten
- Olive oil for cooking

- 2 teaspoons Dijon mustard
- 2 cloves garlic, minced
- Salt and pepper to taste
- Almond-crusted chicken, sliced

Instructions:

1. Preheat the oven to 375°F (190°C).

2. In a shallow dish, combine almond flour, dried oregano, garlic powder, salt, and pepper.

3. Dip each chicken breast into the beaten eggs, coating both sides.

4. Press the egg-coated chicken breasts into the almond flour mixture, ensuring an even coating.

5. In an oven-safe skillet, heat olive oil over medium heat. Cook the chicken breasts for 2-3 minutes on each side until golden brown.

6. Transfer the skillet to the preheated oven and bake for an additional 12-15 minutes or until the chicken is cooked through.

7. In a large bowl, combine chopped romaine lettuce, halved cherry tomatoes, and shaved Parmesan cheese.

8. In a small bowl, whisk together extra-virgin olive oil, lemon juice, Dijon mustard, minced garlic, salt, and pepper to create the dressing.

9. Pour the dressing over the salad and toss to coat evenly.

10. Top the salad with slices of almond-crusted chicken.

Nutritional Information (per serving):

- Carbs: 15g
- Sodium: 300mg

- Fats: 25g
- Protein: 30g

<u>Coconut-Curry Cashew Chicken</u>

Prep Time: 15 minutes | Cook Time: 20 minutes | Servings: 4

Ingredients:

- 1.5 pounds boneless, skinless chicken breasts, cut into cubes
- 1 cup unsalted cashews
- 1 red bell pepper, sliced
- 1 yellow bell pepper, sliced
- 1 onion, thinly sliced
- 3 cloves garlic, minced
- 1 can (13.5 oz) coconut milk
- 2 tablespoons coconut oil
- 2 tablespoons curry powder
- 1 teaspoon ground turmeric
- 1 teaspoon ground ginger
- 1/2 teaspoon cayenne pepper (optional for added heat)
- Salt and pepper to taste
- Fresh cilantro for garnish
- Cooked brown rice for serving

Instructions:

1. In a large skillet, heat coconut oil over medium-high heat.
2. Add cubed chicken to the skillet and cook until browned on all sides.
3. Add sliced red bell pepper, sliced yellow bell pepper, thinly sliced onion, and minced garlic to the skillet. Sauté until the vegetables are tender.
4. Sprinkle curry powder, ground turmeric, ground ginger, and cayenne pepper (if using) over the chicken and vegetables. Stir to coat evenly.
5. Pour in the coconut milk and bring the mixture to a simmer. Allow it to simmer for 10-15 minutes until the chicken is cooked through.
6. Season with salt and pepper to taste.
7. Stir in unsalted cashews and cook for an additional 2-3 minutes until the cashews are heated through.
8. Serve the Coconut-Curry Cashew Chicken over cooked brown rice.
9. Garnish with fresh cilantro before serving.

Nutritional Information (per serving):

- Carbs: 20g
- Sodium: 200mg
- Fats: 25g
- Protein: 30g

Avocado and Blueberry Spinach Salad with Hemp Seeds

Prep Time: 15 minutes | Cook Time: 0 minutes | Servings: 4

Ingredients:

- 8 cups fresh spinach leaves
- 2 avocados, sliced
- 1 cup blueberries
- 1/2 cup red onion, thinly sliced
- 1/4 cup hemp seeds
- 1/4 cup extra-virgin olive oil
- 2 tablespoons balsamic vinegar
- 1 teaspoon Dijon mustard
- Salt and pepper to taste

Instructions:

1. In a large bowl, combine fresh spinach leaves, sliced avocados, blueberries, thinly sliced red onion, and hemp seeds.

2. In a small bowl, whisk together extra-virgin olive oil, balsamic vinegar, Dijon mustard, salt, and pepper to create the dressing.

3. Pour the dressing over the salad and toss gently to coat the ingredients evenly.

4. Divide the salad into individual meal prep containers.

5. Optionally, store the dressing separately to maintain the salad's freshness.

Nutritional Information (per serving):

- Carbs: 15g
- Sodium: 100mg
- Fats: 20g
- Protein: 5g

Chapter 8: Turmeric Infusions

Turmeric-Ginger Lentil Soup

Prep Time: 15 minutes | Cook Time: 30 minutes | Servings: 6

Ingredients:

- 1 cup dried brown lentils, rinsed and drained
- 1 large onion, finely chopped
- 3 carrots, peeled and sliced
- 3 celery stalks, diced
- 3 cloves garlic, minced
- 1 tablespoon fresh ginger, grated
- 1 tablespoon ground turmeric
- 1 teaspoon ground cumin
- 1 teaspoon ground coriander
- 6 cups low-sodium vegetable broth
- 1 can (14 oz) diced tomatoes, undrained
- 1 cup kale, stems removed and chopped
- Salt and pepper to taste
- 2 tablespoons olive oil

Instructions:

1. **Prepare Lentils:** Place the rinsed lentils in a bowl and cover with water. Let them soak while you prepare the other ingredients.

2. **Sauté Vegetables:** In a large pot, heat olive oil over medium heat. Add chopped onions, carrots, and celery. Sauté until the vegetables are tender, about 5-7 minutes.

3. **Add Aromatics:** Stir in minced garlic and grated ginger. Sauté for an additional 1-2 minutes until fragrant.

4. **Season:** Add ground turmeric, cumin, and coriander to the pot. Stir well to coat the vegetables in the spices.

5. **Simmer Soup:** Drain the soaked lentils and add them to the pot. Pour in the vegetable broth and add diced tomatoes with their juice. Bring the soup to a boil, then reduce heat to low, cover, and simmer for 20 minutes or until lentils are tender.

6. **Add Kale:** Stir in chopped kale and continue to simmer for an additional 5 minutes until the kale is wilted.

7. **Season to Taste:** Season the soup with salt and pepper according to your taste preferences.

8. **Serve or Store:** Ladle the soup into bowls and serve immediately, or let it cool for storage. This soup is suitable for meal prep and can be stored in airtight containers in the refrigerator for up to 4 days.

Nutritional Information (per serving):

- Carbs: 32g
- Sodium: 310mg
- Fats: 5g
- Protein: 12g

Turmeric-Cashew Chicken Skewers

Prep Time: 20 minutes | Cook Time: 15 minutes | Servings: 4

Ingredients:

- 1.5 pounds boneless, skinless chicken breasts, cut into 1-inch cubes
- 1/2 cup cashews, finely chopped
- 3 tablespoons olive oil
- 2 tablespoons ground turmeric
- 1 tablespoon smoked paprika
- 2 teaspoons ground cumin
- 3 cloves garlic, minced
- 1 tablespoon honey
- 1 tablespoon apple cider vinegar
- Salt and pepper to taste
- Wooden skewers, soaked in water

Instructions:

1. **Prepare Skewers:** Preheat the grill or grill pan. If using wooden skewers, soak them in water for at least 30 minutes to prevent burning.

2. **Marinate Chicken:** In a bowl, combine olive oil, ground turmeric, smoked paprika, ground cumin, minced garlic, honey, apple cider vinegar, salt, and pepper. Mix well to form a marinade. Add the chicken cubes to the marinade, ensuring they are evenly coated. Allow the chicken to marinate for at least 15 minutes.

3. **Thread Skewers:** Thread marinated chicken cubes onto the soaked wooden skewers, alternating with chopped cashews.

4. **Grill Skewers:** Grill the skewers over medium-high heat for about 6-8 minutes per side or until the chicken is cooked through and has a nice char.

5. **Serve or Store:** Serve the Turmeric-Cashew Chicken Skewers immediately, or let them cool for meal prep. These skewers can be stored in the refrigerator for up to 3 days.

Nutritional Information (per serving):

- Carbs: 12g
- Sodium: 180mg
- Fats: 15g
- Protein: 30g

Golden Turmeric Cauliflower Rice

Prep Time: 15 minutes | Cook Time: 20 minutes | Servings: 4

Ingredients:

- 1 large head of cauliflower, grated
- 1 tablespoon olive oil
- 1 medium onion, finely diced
- 2 cloves garlic, minced
- 1 teaspoon ground turmeric
- 1/2 teaspoon ground ginger
- 1/2 teaspoon ground cumin
- 1/2 teaspoon ground coriander
- 1/4 teaspoon black pepper
- 1/4 cup golden raisins
- 1/4 cup chopped fresh cilantro
- 1/4 cup sliced almonds, toasted

Instructions:

1. Grate the cauliflower using a box grater or pulse in a food processor until it resembles rice. Set aside.
2. In a large skillet, heat olive oil over medium heat.
3. Add finely diced onion and sauté until translucent.
4. Stir in minced garlic and cook for an additional minute until fragrant.
5. Sprinkle ground turmeric, ground ginger, ground cumin, ground coriander, and black pepper over the onion and garlic mixture.
6. Stir well to coat the aromatics with the spices.
7. Add the grated cauliflower to the skillet, stirring to combine with the spiced onion mixture.
8. Cook for 8-10 minutes, stirring occasionally, until the cauliflower rice is tender but not mushy.
9. Mix in golden raisins and chopped fresh cilantro, allowing the flavors to meld for an additional 2-3 minutes.
10. In a separate dry pan, toast sliced almonds over medium heat until golden brown.
11. Transfer the golden turmeric cauliflower rice to serving plates.
12. Garnish with toasted sliced almonds.

Nutritional Information (per serving):

- **Carbs:** 18g
- **Sodium:** 30mg
- **Fats:** 7g
- **Protein:** 5g

Turmeric-Coconut Milk Smoothie Bowl

Prep Time: 10 minutes | Cook Time: 0 minutes | Servings: 2

Ingredients:

- 1 cup frozen mango chunks
- 1 cup frozen pineapple chunks
- 1 banana, sliced
- 1 cup coconut milk (unsweetened)
- 1 teaspoon ground turmeric
- 1/2 teaspoon ground cinnamon
- 1 tablespoon chia seeds
- 2 tablespoons unsweetened shredded coconut
- Fresh berries for garnish
- Mint leaves for garnish

Instructions:

1. Ensure the mango chunks, pineapple chunks, and banana slices are frozen.
2. In a blender, combine frozen mango chunks, frozen pineapple chunks, sliced banana, coconut milk, ground turmeric, and ground cinnamon.
3. Blend until smooth and creamy.
4. Pour the smoothie into two bowls.
5. Sprinkle chia seeds and unsweetened shredded coconut over the smoothie bowls.
6. Top with fresh berries and mint leaves for added flavor and antioxidants.
7. Enjoy the smoothie bowl immediately for a refreshing treat.
8. If meal prepping, store the smoothie base and toppings separately in airtight containers in the refrigerator for up to 24 hours.

Nutritional Information (per serving):

- **Carbs:** 45g
- **Sodium:** 20mg
- **Fats:** 15g
- **Protein:** 5g

Turmeric and Cumin Roasted Carrots

Prep Time: 10 minutes | Cook Time: 25 minutes | Servings: 4

Ingredients:

- 1 pound baby carrots, washed and dried
- 2 tablespoons olive oil
- 1 teaspoon ground turmeric
- 1 teaspoon ground cumin
- 1/2 teaspoon garlic powder
- 1/2 teaspoon onion powder
- Salt and pepper to taste
- Fresh parsley, chopped, for garnish

Instructions:

1. Preheat the oven to 400°F (200°C).
2. Wash and thoroughly dry the baby carrots.
3. In a large bowl, toss the baby carrots with olive oil, ensuring they are well-coated.
4. Sprinkle ground turmeric, ground cumin, garlic powder, onion powder, salt, and pepper over the carrots.
5. Toss again to evenly distribute the seasonings.
6. Spread the seasoned carrots in a single layer on a baking sheet.
7. Roast in the preheated oven for 20-25 minutes or until the carrots are tender and slightly caramelized, stirring halfway through.
8. Remove from the oven and transfer the roasted carrots to a serving dish.
9. Garnish with freshly chopped parsley.
10. Enjoy the roasted carrots immediately as a side dish.
11. For meal prep, let them cool completely before storing in airtight containers in the refrigerator for up to 3 days.

Nutritional Information (per serving):

- **Carbs:** 10g
- **Sodium:** 80mg
- **Fats:** 7g
- **Protein:** 1g

<u>Creamy Turmeric Chicken and Broccoli Casserole</u>

Prep Time: 15 minutes | Cook Time: 30 minutes | Servings: 6

Ingredients:

- 1.5 pounds boneless, skinless chicken breasts, diced
- 4 cups broccoli florets, blanched
- 2 cups brown rice, cooked
- 1 cup Greek yogurt
- 1 cup low-sodium chicken broth
- 1/2 cup unsweetened almond milk
- 1/4 cup olive oil
- 3 tablespoons all-purpose flour
- 2 teaspoons ground turmeric
- 1 teaspoon garlic powder
- 1 teaspoon onion powder
- Salt and pepper to taste
- 1/2 cup grated Parmesan cheese
- Fresh parsley, chopped, for garnish

Instructions:

1. Preheat the oven to 375°F (190°C).
2. In a large skillet, heat olive oil over medium heat.
3. Add diced chicken and cook until browned and cooked through.
4. Sprinkle flour over the cooked chicken and stir to create a roux.
5. Incorporate ground turmeric, garlic powder, onion powder, salt, and pepper into the roux, stirring to combine.
6. Gradually add chicken broth and almond milk, stirring continuously until the mixture thickens.
7. Remove the skillet from heat and fold in Greek yogurt until well combined.
8. In a large mixing bowl, combine blanched broccoli, cooked brown rice, and the creamy turmeric chicken mixture.
9. Transfer the mixture to a greased casserole dish.
10. Sprinkle grated Parmesan cheese over the casserole.
11. Bake in the preheated oven for 20-25 minutes or until the casserole is bubbly and golden.
12. Remove from the oven, garnish with chopped fresh parsley, and serve.
13. Enjoy the casserole immediately or let it cool before storing in airtight containers in the refrigerator for up to 3 days.

Nutritional Information (per serving):

- **Carbs:** 32g
- **Sodium:** 180mg
- **Fats:** 16g
- **Protein:** 30g

Turmeric-Spiced Quinoa Patties

Prep Time: 20 minutes | Cook Time: 20 minutes | Servings: 4

Ingredients:

- 1 cup quinoa, cooked and cooled
- 1 can (15 ounces) chickpeas, drained and rinsed
- 1 cup spinach, finely chopped
- 1/2 cup red bell pepper, finely diced
- 1/4 cup red onion, finely chopped
- 2 cloves garlic, minced
- 1 teaspoon ground turmeric
- 1/2 teaspoon ground cumin
- 1/2 teaspoon paprika
- 1/4 teaspoon cayenne pepper (optional)
- Salt and pepper to taste
- 2 large eggs, beaten
- 1/4 cup whole wheat breadcrumbs
- 2 tablespoons olive oil, for cooking

Instructions:

1. Cook quinoa according to package instructions. Allow it to cool.
2. In a food processor, pulse chickpeas until coarsely ground.
3. In a large mixing bowl, combine cooked and cooled quinoa, ground chickpeas, chopped spinach, diced red bell pepper, chopped red onion, minced garlic, ground turmeric, ground cumin, paprika, cayenne pepper (if using), salt, and pepper.
4. Mix in beaten eggs and whole wheat breadcrumbs to bind the mixture.
5. Divide the mixture into 8 portions and shape them into patties.
6. In a large skillet, heat olive oil over medium heat.
7. Cook the quinoa patties for about 4-5 minutes per side or until golden brown and cooked through.
8. Serve the turmeric-spiced quinoa patties immediately.
9. For meal prep, let them cool before storing in airtight containers in the refrigerator for up to 3 days.

Nutritional Information (per serving):

- **Carbs:** 38g
- **Sodium:** 250mg
- **Fats:** 11g
- **Protein:** 14g

Golden Milk Chia Pudding Parfait

Prep Time: 15 minutes (+ chilling time) | Cook Time: 0 minutes | Servings: 4

Ingredients:

For Chia Pudding:

- 1/2 cup chia seeds
- 2 cups unsweetened almond milk
- 1 teaspoon ground turmeric
- 1/2 teaspoon ground cinnamon
- 1/4 teaspoon ground ginger
- 1/4 teaspoon cardamom
- 2 tablespoons maple syrup (optional)

For Parfait:

- 2 cups Greek yogurt (unsweetened)
- 1 cup mixed berries (blueberries, raspberries, strawberries)
- 1/4 cup unsweetened shredded coconut
- 1/4 cup chopped almonds, toasted
- Fresh mint leaves for garnish

Instructions:

1. In a bowl, whisk together chia seeds, almond milk, ground turmeric, ground cinnamon, ground ginger, cardamom, and maple syrup (if using).
2. Let it sit for 5 minutes, whisking occasionally to avoid clumps.
3. Cover and refrigerate for at least 4 hours or overnight until the chia pudding thickens.
4. In serving glasses or jars, layer the chia pudding with unsweetened Greek yogurt.
5. Top the yogurt layer with mixed berries.
6. Sprinkle unsweetened shredded coconut and toasted chopped almonds over the berries.
7. Repeat the layers until the glasses or jars are filled.
8. Garnish with fresh mint leaves.
9. Cover and refrigerate for at least 1 hour before serving.
10. Serve the golden milk chia pudding parfait chilled.
11. For meal prep, cover tightly and store in the refrigerator for up to 3 days.

Nutritional Information (per serving):

- **Carbs:** 30g
- **Sodium:** 80mg
- **Fats:** 15g
- **Protein:** 15g

<u>Turmeric-Lemon Grilled Chicken Thighs</u>

Prep Time: 15 minutes (+ marinating time) | Cook Time: 20 minutes | Servings: 4

Ingredients:

- 8 bone-in, skin-on chicken thighs
- 1/4 cup olive oil
- Zest and juice of 2 lemons
- 2 teaspoons ground turmeric
- 1 teaspoon smoked paprika
- 1 teaspoon garlic powder
- 1 teaspoon onion powder
- Salt and pepper to taste
- Fresh parsley, chopped, for garnish

Instructions:

1. In a bowl, whisk together olive oil, lemon zest, lemon juice, ground turmeric, smoked paprika, garlic powder, onion powder, salt, and pepper.
2. Place chicken thighs in a resealable plastic bag or a shallow dish. Pour the marinade over the chicken, ensuring even coating. Marinate in the refrigerator for at least 1 hour, or preferably overnight.
3. Preheat the grill to medium-high heat.
4. Take the chicken thighs out of the marinade, allowing excess to drip off.
5. Place the chicken thighs on the preheated grill. Grill for approximately 10 minutes per side or until the internal temperature reaches 165°F (74°C) and the skin is crispy.
6. Remove the grilled chicken thighs from the grill and let them rest for a few minutes.
7. Garnish with freshly chopped parsley.
8. Serve the turmeric-lemon grilled chicken thighs immediately.
9. For meal prep, let the chicken cool before storing in airtight containers in the refrigerator for up to 3 days.

Nutritional Information (per serving):

- **Carbs:** 0g
- **Sodium:** 80mg
- **Fats:** 20g
- **Protein:** 32g

<u>Turmeric-Carrot Muffins with Coconut Glaze</u>

Prep Time: 20 minutes | Cook Time: 20 minutes | Servings: 12

Ingredients:

For Muffins:

- 2 cups whole wheat flour
- 1 teaspoon baking powder
- 1/2 teaspoon baking soda
- 1/2 teaspoon ground turmeric
- 1/2 teaspoon ground cinnamon
- 1/4 teaspoon ground ginger
- 1/4 teaspoon salt
- 1 cup grated carrots
- 1/2 cup unsweetened applesauce
- 1/2 cup maple syrup
- 1/4 cup olive oil
- 2 large eggs
- 1 teaspoon vanilla extract

For Coconut Glaze:

- 1/2 cup coconut cream
- 2 tablespoons maple syrup
- Shredded coconut for garnish

Instructions:

1. Preheat the oven to 350°F (175°C). Line a muffin tin with paper liners.
2. In a bowl, whisk together whole wheat flour, baking powder, baking soda, ground turmeric, ground cinnamon, ground ginger, and salt.
3. In another bowl, combine grated carrots, unsweetened applesauce, maple syrup, olive oil, eggs, and vanilla extract.
4. Pour the wet ingredients into the dry ingredients. Mix until just combined. Do not overmix.
5. Divide the batter evenly among the muffin cups, filling each about two-thirds full.
6. Bake for 18-20 minutes or until a toothpick inserted into the center comes out clean.
7. Allow the muffins to cool in the tin for 5 minutes, then transfer them to a wire rack to cool completely.
8. In a small saucepan, heat coconut cream and maple syrup over low heat until well combined. Let it cool slightly.
9. Drizzle the coconut glaze over the cooled muffins.
10. Garnish with shredded coconut.
11. Serve the turmeric-carrot muffins immediately or store them in an airtight container at room temperature for up to 3 days.

Nutritional Information (per serving):

- **Carbs:** 27g
- **Sodium:** 120mg
- **Fats:** 8g
- **Protein:** 3g

<u>Coconut Turmeric Shrimp Stir-Fry</u>

Prep Time: 15 minutes | Cook Time: 10 minutes | Servings: 4

Ingredients:

- 1 pound large shrimp, peeled and deveined
- 2 tablespoons coconut oil
- 1 onion, thinly sliced
- 2 bell peppers (1 red, 1 yellow), thinly sliced
- 1 cup snap peas, ends trimmed
- 3 cloves garlic, minced
- 1 tablespoon fresh ginger, grated
- 1 teaspoon ground turmeric
- 1/2 teaspoon ground coriander
- 1/2 teaspoon paprika
- 1 can (14 ounces) coconut milk
- Salt and pepper to taste
- Fresh cilantro for garnish
- Cooked brown rice for serving

Instructions:

1. Ensure shrimp are peeled and deveined.
2. In a large wok or skillet, heat coconut oil over medium-high heat.
3. Add thinly sliced onion and bell peppers to the wok. Stir-fry for 2-3 minutes until slightly softened.
4. Add snap peas to the wok and continue to stir-fry for an additional 2 minutes.
5. Stir in minced garlic and grated fresh ginger. Sauté for 1 minute until fragrant.
6. Add the peeled and deveined shrimp to the wok. Cook until shrimp turn pink and opaque, approximately 2-3 minutes.
7. Sprinkle ground turmeric, ground coriander, and paprika over the shrimp and vegetables. Stir to coat evenly.
8. Pour in the coconut milk, stirring well to combine all ingredients. Simmer for 2-3 minutes.
9. Season the stir-fry with salt and pepper to taste. Adjust accordingly.
10. Garnish with fresh cilantro.
11. Serve the coconut turmeric shrimp stir-fry over cooked brown rice.
12. Serve immediately or store in airtight containers in the refrigerator for up to 2 days.

Nutritional Information (per serving):

- **Carbs:** 20g
- **Sodium:** 250mg
- **Fats:** 18g
- **Protein:** 25g

Turmeric and Coriander Roasted Chickpeas

Prep Time: 10 minutes | Cook Time: 30 minutes | Servings: 4

Ingredients:

- 2 cans (15 ounces each) chickpeas, drained and rinsed
- 2 tablespoons olive oil
- 1 teaspoon ground turmeric
- 1 teaspoon ground coriander
- 1/2 teaspoon cumin
- 1/2 teaspoon smoked paprika
- 1/4 teaspoon cayenne pepper (optional)
- Salt and pepper to taste
- Fresh cilantro, chopped, for garnish

Instructions:

- Preheat the oven to 400°F (200°C).
- Drain and rinse the chickpeas. Pat them dry with a paper towel to remove excess moisture.
- In a bowl, toss the dried chickpeas with olive oil, ground turmeric, ground coriander, cumin, smoked paprika, cayenne pepper (if using), salt, and pepper.
- Spread the seasoned chickpeas in a single layer on a baking sheet.
- Roast in the preheated oven for 25-30 minutes, shaking the pan occasionally for even cooking. The chickpeas should become golden and crispy.
- Allow the roasted chickpeas to cool slightly. Sprinkle fresh cilantro over the top for added flavor.
- Serve the turmeric and coriander roasted chickpeas as a snack or salad topper.
- For meal prep, let them cool completely before storing in airtight containers. They can be stored at room temperature for up to a week.

Nutritional Information (per serving):

- **Carbs:** 29g
- **Sodium:** 320mg
- **Fats:** 8g
- **Protein:** 11g

<u>Mango-Turmeric Lassi with Mint</u>

Prep Time: 10 minutes | Cook Time: 0 minutes | Servings: 2

Ingredients:

- 1 cup ripe mango, peeled and diced
- 1 cup plain Greek yogurt (unsweetened)
- 1/2 cup cold water
- 1/2 teaspoon ground turmeric
- 1 tablespoon honey (optional)
- Fresh mint leaves for garnish
- Ice cubes (optional)

Instructions:

1. Peel and dice ripe mango.
2. In a blender, combine diced mango, plain Greek yogurt, cold water, ground turmeric, and honey (if using). Blend until smooth and creamy.
3. Taste the lassi and add more honey if additional sweetness is desired. Blend again if necessary.
4. Refrigerate the lassi for at least 30 minutes to enhance flavors. You can also add ice cubes for immediate serving.
5. Pour the mango-turmeric lassi into glasses.
6. Garnish with fresh mint leaves.
7. Serve the lassi immediately for a refreshing drink.
8. For meal prep, store the lassi in airtight containers in the refrigerator for up to 24 hours.

Nutritional Information (per serving):

- **Carbs:** 30g
- **Sodium:** 50mg
- **Fats:** 1g
- **Protein:** 11g

Turmeric and Basil Zucchini Noodles

Prep Time: 15 minutes | Cook Time: 5 minutes | Servings: 4

Ingredients:

- 4 medium zucchinis, spiralized
- 2 tablespoons olive oil
- 3 cloves garlic, minced
- 1 teaspoon ground turmeric
- 1/2 teaspoon red pepper flakes (optional)
- Salt and pepper to taste
- 1/4 cup fresh basil, thinly sliced
- 1 tablespoon lemon juice
- Grated Parmesan cheese for garnish (optional)

Instructions:

1. Spiralize the zucchinis into noodle-like shapes.
2. In a large skillet, heat olive oil over medium heat. Add minced garlic and sauté until fragrant.
3. Add the spiralized zucchini noodles to the skillet. Toss and cook for 2-3 minutes until just tender. Avoid overcooking to maintain a slight crunch.
4. Sprinkle ground turmeric and red pepper flakes (if using) over the zucchini noodles. Toss to evenly coat.
5. Season the noodles with salt and pepper to taste. Adjust according to your preference.
6. Stir in thinly sliced fresh basil. Reserve some for garnish if desired.
7. Drizzle lemon juice over the zucchini noodles. Toss once more to combine.
8. Garnish with additional fresh basil and grated Parmesan cheese if desired.
9. Serve the turmeric and basil zucchini noodles immediately.
10. For meal prep, let them cool before storing in airtight containers in the refrigerator for up to 2 days.

Nutritional Information (per serving):

- **Carbs:** 7g
- **Sodium:** 30mg
- **Fats:** 5g
- **Protein:** 2g

Turmeric-Spiced Sweet Potato Soup

Prep Time: 15 minutes | Cook Time: 30 minutes | Servings: 6

Ingredients:

- 2 tablespoons olive oil
- 1 onion, diced
- 3 cloves garlic, minced
- 1 tablespoon fresh ginger, grated
- 2 teaspoons ground turmeric
- 1/2 teaspoon ground cinnamon
- 1/4 teaspoon ground nutmeg
- 3 large sweet potatoes, peeled and diced
- 4 cups vegetable broth (low-sodium)
- 1 can (14 ounces) coconut milk (unsweetened)
- Salt and pepper to taste
- Fresh cilantro, chopped, for garnish

Instructions:

1. In a large pot, heat olive oil over medium heat. Add diced onion, minced garlic, and grated fresh ginger. Sauté until the onion is translucent.
2. Sprinkle ground turmeric, ground cinnamon, and ground nutmeg over the sautéed aromatics. Stir to coat.
3. Add diced sweet potatoes to the pot. Mix well to combine with the aromatics and spices.
4. Pour in low-sodium vegetable broth. Bring the mixture to a boil, then reduce the heat and let it simmer until the sweet potatoes are tender.
5. Use an immersion blender to puree the soup until smooth. Alternatively, transfer the mixture to a blender in batches, blending until smooth. Exercise caution when blending hot liquids.
6. Pour in unsweetened coconut milk, stirring well to combine. Simmer for an additional 5 minutes.
7. Season the soup with salt and pepper to taste. Adjust according to your preference.
8. Garnish the turmeric-spiced sweet potato soup with chopped fresh cilantro.
9. Serve the soup immediately or let it cool before storing in airtight containers. Refrigerate for up to 3 days.

Nutritional Information (per serving):

- **Carbs:** 30g
- **Sodium:** 180mg
- **Fats:** 9g
- **Protein:** 3g

Grilled Turmeric Tofu Skewers

Prep Time: 30 minutes (plus marinating time) | Cook Time: 10 minutes | Servings: 4

Ingredients:

- 1 block (14 ounces) extra-firm tofu, pressed and cubed
- 2 tablespoons olive oil
- 2 teaspoons ground turmeric
- 1 teaspoon ground cumin
- 1 teaspoon paprika
- 1 teaspoon garlic powder
- 1/2 teaspoon cayenne pepper (optional)
- Salt and pepper to taste
- Wooden skewers, soaked in water

Instructions:

- Press the tofu to remove excess moisture, then cut it into cubes.
- In a bowl, whisk together olive oil, ground turmeric, ground cumin, paprika, garlic powder, cayenne pepper (if using), salt, and pepper.
- Place the tofu cubes in a shallow dish and pour the marinade over them. Ensure each piece is well-coated. Marinate for at least 30 minutes, or preferably overnight in the refrigerator.
- Preheat the grill to medium-high heat.
- Thread the marinated tofu cubes onto soaked wooden skewers. Leave a little space between each piece.
- Grill the tofu skewers for about 4-5 minutes per side or until they develop grill marks and are heated through.
- Periodically baste the tofu skewers with the remaining marinade during grilling for added flavor.
- Serve the grilled turmeric tofu skewers immediately.
- For meal prep, let them cool before storing in airtight containers in the refrigerator for up to 3 days.

Nutritional Information (per serving):

- **Carbs:** 2g
- **Sodium:** 80mg
- **Fats:** 15g
- **Protein:** 10g

Turmeric and Cinnamon Baked Apples

Prep Time: 15 minutes | Cook Time: 30 minutes | Servings: 4

Ingredients:

- 4 large apples, cored and sliced
- 2 tablespoons coconut oil, melted
- 1 teaspoon ground turmeric
- 1 teaspoon ground cinnamon
- 1/4 teaspoon ground nutmeg
- 1/4 teaspoon ground ginger
- 1 tablespoon honey or maple syrup (optional)
- Chopped nuts for garnish (optional)

Instructions:

1. Preheat the oven to 375°F (190°C).
2. Core and slice the apples. Leave the skin on for added nutrients.
3. In a bowl, combine melted coconut oil, ground turmeric, ground cinnamon, ground nutmeg, and ground ginger. Mix well to create a coating.
4. Place the sliced apples in the bowl with the turmeric-cinnamon coating. Toss until the apples are evenly coated.
5. Transfer the coated apples to a baking dish, spreading them out into an even layer.
6. If desired, drizzle honey or maple syrup over the apples for added sweetness. This step is optional.
7. Bake in the preheated oven for approximately 30 minutes or until the apples are tender, stirring halfway through the baking time.
8. If desired, garnish the baked apples with chopped nuts for added texture.
9. Serve the turmeric and cinnamon baked apples warm.
10. For meal prep, let them cool before storing in airtight containers in the refrigerator for up to 3 days.

Nutritional Information (per serving):

- **Carbs:** 25g
- **Sodium:** 0mg
- **Fats:** 7g
- **Protein:** 0g

<u>Turmeric-Lime Coconut Energy Bites</u>

Prep Time: 20 minutes | Cook Time: 0 minutes | Servings: 12

Ingredients:

- 1 cup old-fashioned oats
- 1/2 cup unsweetened shredded coconut
- 1/2 cup almond butter
- 1/4 cup honey or maple syrup
- Zest of 1 lime
- 2 tablespoons chia seeds
- 1 teaspoon ground turmeric
- 1/2 teaspoon vanilla extract
- Pinch of salt
- Extra shredded coconut for coating (optional)

Instructions:

1. Gather all the ingredients.
2. In a large bowl, combine old-fashioned oats, unsweetened shredded coconut, chia seeds, ground turmeric, and a pinch of salt.
3. Add almond butter, honey or maple syrup, lime zest, and vanilla extract to the dry ingredients.
4. Mix all the ingredients thoroughly until well combined. The mixture should be sticky and easily moldable.
5. Take about a tablespoon of the mixture and roll it between your palms to form a ball. Repeat until all the mixture is used.
6. If desired, roll the energy bites in extra shredded coconut to coat the exterior.
7. Place the energy bites in the refrigerator for at least 1 hour to firm up.
8. Serve the turmeric-lime coconut energy bites chilled.
9. For meal prep, store in an airtight container in the refrigerator for up to 1 week.

Nutritional Information (per serving, 1 energy bite):

- **Carbs:** 11g
- **Sodium:** 10mg
- **Fats:** 7g
- **Protein:** 3g

Chapter 9: Berry Bliss

Mixed Berry and Almond Overnight Oats

Prep Time: 10 minutes | **Cook Time:** 0 minutes | **Servings:** 4

Ingredients:

- 2 cups old-fashioned rolled oats

- 2 cups unsweetened almond milk

- 1 cup mixed berries (blueberries, strawberries, raspberries)

- 1/2 cup sliced almonds

- 4 tablespoons chia seeds

- 4 tablespoons pure maple syrup

- 1 teaspoon vanilla extract

- 1/2 teaspoon ground cinnamon

- Pinch of sea salt

Nutritional Information (per serving):

- **Carbs:** 45g

- **Sodium:** 80mg

- **Fats:** 15g

- **Protein:** 10g

Instructions:

1. In a large bowl, combine the rolled oats, almond milk, chia seeds, maple syrup, vanilla extract, cinnamon, and a pinch of sea salt. Mix well to ensure all ingredients are evenly distributed.

2. Gently fold in the mixed berries and sliced almonds, ensuring they are evenly distributed throughout the mixture.

3. Cover the bowl with a lid or plastic wrap and refrigerate overnight, or for at least 8 hours. This allows the oats and chia seeds to absorb the liquid and create a creamy texture.

4. Before serving, give the overnight oats a good stir to combine all the ingredients. If the mixture is too thick, you can add a splash of almond milk to reach your desired consistency.

5. Divide the mixed berry and almond overnight oats into individual servings.

6. Optionally, garnish with additional berries and sliced almonds before serving.

Grilled Chicken Salad with Berry Vinaigrette

Prep Time: 15 minutes | **Cook Time:** 15 minutes | **Servings:** 4

Ingredients:

For the Salad:

- 1 pound boneless, skinless chicken breasts
- 8 cups mixed salad greens
- 1 cup cherry tomatoes, halved
- 1 cucumber, sliced
- 1/2 red onion, thinly sliced
- 1/2 cup sliced almonds, toasted
- 1/4 cup feta cheese, crumbled (optional)

For the Berry Vinaigrette:

- 1 cup mixed berries (strawberries, blueberries, raspberries)
- 1/4 cup olive oil
- 2 tablespoons balsamic vinegar
- 1 tablespoon honey
- 1 teaspoon Dijon mustard
- Salt and pepper to taste

Nutritional Information (per serving):

- **Carbs:** 20g
- **Sodium:** 120mg
- **Fats:** 15g
- **Protein:** 25g

Instructions:

1. Preheat the grill to medium-high heat.
2. Season the chicken breasts with salt and pepper.
3. Grill the chicken for about 6-8 minutes per side or until the internal temperature reaches 165°F (74°C).
4. Allow the chicken to rest for 5 minutes before slicing it into thin strips.
5. In a large bowl, combine the mixed salad greens, cherry tomatoes, sliced cucumber, red onion, and toasted sliced almonds. Add the crumbled feta cheese if desired.
6. In a blender, combine the mixed berries, olive oil, balsamic vinegar, honey, Dijon mustard, salt, and pepper.
7. Blend until smooth and well combined.
8. Distribute the grilled chicken strips over the prepared salad.
9. Drizzle the berry vinaigrette over the grilled chicken salad just before serving.
10. Choose extra-virgin olive oil for its anti-inflammatory properties.
11. Opt for fresh berries, as they contain more antioxidants.
12. Limit the amount of added salt and consider omitting the feta cheese to reduce sodium content.
13. Include turmeric or ginger in the vinaigrette for an extra anti-inflammatory boost.

<u>Quinoa and Berry Stuffed Bell Peppers</u>

Prep Time: 20 minutes | **Cook Time:** 25 minutes | **Servings:** 4

Ingredients:

- 4 large bell peppers, halved and seeds removed
- 1 cup quinoa, rinsed
- 2 cups low-sodium vegetable broth
- 1 cup mixed berries (blueberries, raspberries)
- 1 cup spinach, chopped
- 1/2 cup red onion, finely chopped
- 1/2 cup walnuts, chopped
- 2 cloves garlic, minced
- 2 tablespoons olive oil
- 1 teaspoon ground cumin
- 1/2 teaspoon turmeric
- Salt and pepper to taste
- Fresh parsley for garnish (optional)

Nutritional Information (per serving):

- **Carbs:** 40g
- **Sodium:** 80mg
- **Fats:** 15g
- **Protein:** 10g

Instructions:

1. Preheat the oven to 375°F (190°C).
2. In a medium saucepan, bring the vegetable broth to a boil.
3. Add the quinoa, reduce heat to low, cover, and simmer for 15 minutes or until the quinoa is cooked and the liquid is absorbed.
4. In a skillet over medium heat, add olive oil.
5. Add chopped red onion and minced garlic, sauté until softened.
6. Stir in chopped spinach and cook until wilted.
7. In a large bowl, combine cooked quinoa, sautéed vegetables, mixed berries, chopped walnuts, ground cumin, turmeric, salt, and pepper. Mix well.
8. Place the halved bell peppers in a baking dish.
9. Fill each pepper half with the quinoa and berry mixture.
10. Cover the baking dish with foil and bake for 20-25 minutes, or until the peppers are tender.
11. If desired, garnish with fresh parsley before serving.
12. Use low-sodium vegetable broth to reduce sodium content.
13. Incorporate turmeric for its anti-inflammatory properties.
14. Opt for fresh berries, as they contain more antioxidants.
15. Choose heart-healthy olive oil for sautéing.

Berry Chia Seed Jam

Prep Time: 5 minutes | **Cook Time:** 15 minutes | **Servings:** Approximately 16 (2-tablespoon servings)

Ingredients:

- 3 cups mixed berries (strawberries, blueberries, raspberries)
- 3 tablespoons chia seeds
- 2 tablespoons maple syrup
- 1 tablespoon lemon juice
- 1/2 teaspoon vanilla extract
- Pinch of cinnamon
- Pinch of sea salt

Nutritional Information (per 2-tablespoon serving):

- **Carbs:** 6g
- **Sodium:** 10mg
- **Fats:** 2g
- **Protein:** 1g

Instructions:

1. If using strawberries, hull and chop them. Leave blueberries and raspberries whole.
2. In a saucepan over medium heat, combine the mixed berries, maple syrup, lemon juice, vanilla extract, cinnamon, and a pinch of sea salt.
3. Bring the mixture to a simmer, stirring occasionally. Allow the berries to break down and release their juices.
4. Once the berries are softened, stir in the chia seeds. Mix well to combine.
5. Continue to simmer the mixture, stirring frequently, until it thickens to your desired consistency. This usually takes about 10-15 minutes.
6. Taste the jam and adjust sweetness by adding more maple syrup if needed.
7. Remove the saucepan from heat and let the jam cool to room temperature. It will continue to thicken as it cools.
8. Choose fresh berries for their higher antioxidant content.
9. Replace maple syrup with honey for potential anti-inflammatory benefits.
10. Include a pinch of cinnamon for its anti-inflammatory properties.
11. Opt for sea salt instead of table salt to reduce sodium content.
12. Store the berry chia seed jam in sterilized jars with airtight lids.
13. Refrigerate for up to two weeks or freeze for longer storage. Thaw frozen jam in the refrigerator before use.

<u>Mixed Berry and Spinach Smoothie Bowl</u>

Prep Time: 10 minutes | **Cook Time:** 0 minutes | **Servings:** 2

Ingredients:

For the Smoothie Bowl:

- 2 cups mixed berries (strawberries, blueberries, raspberries)
- 1 ripe banana, sliced and frozen
- 2 cups fresh spinach leaves
- 1/2 cup Greek yogurt
-)
- 1/2 cup almond milk (unsweetened)
- 1 tablespoon chia seeds
- 1 tablespoon honey or maple syrup (optional for sweetness

For Toppings:

- Sliced strawberries
- Blueberries
- Granola
- Chopped nuts (almonds, walnuts)

Nutritional Information (per serving):

- **Carbs:** 40g
- **Sodium:** 60mg
- **Fats:** 8g
- **Protein:** 10g

Instructions:

1. Slice and freeze the ripe banana ahead of time.
2. In a blender, combine the mixed berries, frozen banana slices, fresh spinach leaves, Greek yogurt, almond milk, chia seeds, and optional honey or maple syrup.
3. Blend the ingredients until you achieve a smooth and creamy consistency.
4. If the smoothie is too thick, add more almond milk in small increments until you reach your desired thickness.
5. Divide the smoothie mixture into two bowls.
6. Top each smoothie bowl with sliced strawberries, blueberries, granola, and chopped nuts.
7. Choose fresh berries for their higher antioxidant content.
8. Opt for unsweetened almond milk to keep added sugars low.
9. Consider adding a pinch of turmeric or ginger to the smoothie for their potential anti-inflammatory properties.

Berry and Walnut Quinoa Salad

Prep Time: 15 minutes | **Cook Time:** 15 minutes | **Servings:** 4

Ingredients:

- 1 cup quinoa, rinsed
- 2 cups water
- 1 cup mixed berries (blueberries, raspberries)
- 1/2 cup walnuts, chopped
- 1/2 cup cucumber, diced
- 1/4 cup red onion, finely chopped
- 1/4 cup fresh mint leaves, chopped
- 1/4 cup feta cheese, crumbled (optional)

For the Dressing:

- 3 tablespoons extra-virgin olive oil
- 2 tablespoons balsamic vinegar
- 1 tablespoon honey
- 1 teaspoon Dijon mustard
- Salt and pepper to taste

Nutritional Information (per serving):

- **Carbs:** 35g
- **Sodium:** 40mg
- **Fats:** 15g
- **Protein:** 8g

Instructions:

1. In a medium saucepan, combine the quinoa and water. Bring to a boil, then reduce heat to low, cover, and simmer for 15 minutes or until the quinoa is cooked and water is absorbed.
2. In a small bowl, whisk together the olive oil, balsamic vinegar, honey, Dijon mustard, salt, and pepper. Set aside.
3. Fluff the cooked quinoa with a fork and let it cool to room temperature.
4. In a large bowl, combine the cooled quinoa, mixed berries, chopped walnuts, diced cucumber, finely chopped red onion, and chopped fresh mint.
5. If using, add crumbled feta cheese to the salad.
6. Pour the prepared dressing over the salad ingredients.
7. Gently toss the salad until all ingredients are well coated with the dressing.
8. Use extra-virgin olive oil for its anti-inflammatory properties.
9. Choose fresh berries for their higher antioxidant content.
10. Include turmeric or ginger in the dressing for an extra anti-inflammatory boost.
11. Consider omitting or reducing the amount of feta cheese to lower sodium content.

Balsamic Berry Chicken Skewers

Prep Time: 20 minutes | **Cook Time:** 15 minutes | **Servings:** 4

Ingredients:

- 1.5 pounds boneless, skinless chicken breasts, cut into cubes
- 2 cups mixed berries (strawberries, blueberries, raspberries)
- 1 red onion, cut into chunks
- 1/4 cup balsamic vinegar
- 2 tablespoons olive oil
- 2 tablespoons honey
- 2 cloves garlic, minced
- 1 teaspoon dried thyme
- Salt and pepper to taste
- Wooden or metal skewers

Nutritional Information (per serving):

- **Carbs:** 20g
- **Sodium:** 60mg
- **Fats:** 10g
- **Protein:** 30g

Instructions:

1. In a bowl, combine the chicken cubes, balsamic vinegar, olive oil, honey, minced garlic, dried thyme, salt, and pepper. Allow it to marinate for at least 15 minutes.
2. Preheat the grill or oven to medium-high heat.
3. Thread marinated chicken cubes onto skewers, alternating with chunks of red onion and mixed berries.
4. Grill the skewers for about 12-15 minutes, turning occasionally, until the chicken is cooked through and has a nice char.
5. While grilling, baste the skewers with the remaining marinade to enhance flavor.
6. Choose extra-virgin olive oil for its anti-inflammatory properties.
7. Use honey for sweetness, which may have anti-inflammatory benefits.
8. Add minced ginger to the marinade for an extra anti-inflammatory boost.
9. Limit added salt to reduce sodium content.

Berry Avocado Salsa with Cinnamon Tortilla Chips

Prep Time: 15 minutes | **Cook Time:** 10 minutes | **Servings:** 6

Ingredients:

For the Berry Avocado Salsa:

- 1 cup strawberries, diced
- 1 cup blueberries
- 1 cup raspberries
- 1 ripe avocado, diced
- 1/4 cup red onion, finely chopped
- 1/4 cup fresh mint leaves, chopped
- 1 tablespoon balsamic vinegar
- 1 tablespoon extra-virgin olive oil
- 1 teaspoon honey
- Salt to taste

For the Cinnamon Tortilla Chips:

- 6 whole wheat or multigrain tortillas
- 2 tablespoons olive oil
- 1 tablespoon ground cinnamon
- 1 tablespoon sugar (optional)

Nutritional Information (per serving):

- **Carbs:** 30g
- **Sodium:** 80mg
- **Fats:** 10g
- **Protein:** 3g

Instructions:

1. Preheat the oven to 350°F (175°C).
2. In a bowl, combine diced strawberries, blueberries, raspberries, diced avocado, finely chopped red onion, and chopped fresh mint leaves.
3. In a separate small bowl, whisk together balsamic vinegar, extra-virgin olive oil, honey, and a pinch of salt.
4. Pour the dressing over the berry and avocado mixture. Gently toss until well combined. Refrigerate while preparing the cinnamon tortilla chips.
5. Brush both sides of each tortilla with olive oil.
6. In a small bowl, mix ground cinnamon with sugar (if using).
7. Sprinkle the cinnamon mixture over the tortillas.
8. Stack the tortillas and cut them into wedges.
9. Arrange the tortilla wedges in a single layer on a baking sheet.
10. Bake for 8-10 minutes or until the chips are golden and crispy.
11. Choose whole wheat or multigrain tortillas for added fiber and anti-inflammatory benefits.
12. Use extra-virgin olive oil for its anti-inflammatory properties.
13. Include honey for sweetness, which may have anti-inflammatory benefits.
14. Limit added salt to reduce sodium content.
15. Allow the cinnamon tortilla chips to cool before serving with the chilled berry avocado salsa.

Raspberry and Almond Baked Salmon

Prep Time: 15 minutes | **Cook Time:** 20 minutes | **Servings:** 4

Ingredients:

- 4 salmon fillets
- 1 cup fresh raspberries
- 1/2 cup sliced almonds
- 2 tablespoons olive oil
- 2 tablespoons balsamic vinegar
- 1 tablespoon honey
- 1 tablespoon Dijon mustard
- 2 cloves garlic, minced
- Salt and pepper to taste
- Fresh parsley for garnish (optional)

Nutritional Information (per serving):

- **Carbs:** 10g
- **Sodium:** 60mg
- **Fats:** 20g
- **Protein:** 25g

Instructions:

1. Preheat the oven to 400°F (200°C).
2. In a bowl, combine fresh raspberries and sliced almonds.
3. In a small bowl, whisk together olive oil, balsamic vinegar, honey, Dijon mustard, minced garlic, salt, and pepper.
4. Place the salmon fillets on a parchment-lined baking sheet.
5. Spoon the raspberry and almond mixture evenly over the salmon fillets.
6. Drizzle the balsamic honey glaze over the raspberry and almond-topped salmon.
7. Bake in the preheated oven for approximately 15-20 minutes or until the salmon is cooked through and flakes easily with a fork.
8. If desired, garnish with fresh parsley before serving.
9. Use extra-virgin olive oil for its anti-inflammatory properties.
10. Incorporate honey for sweetness, which may have anti-inflammatory benefits.
11. Include garlic for its potential anti-inflammatory effects.
12. Limit added salt to reduce sodium content.

Blueberry and Kale Salad with Lemon Poppyseed Dressing

Prep Time: 15 minutes | **Cook Time:** 0 minutes | **Servings:** 4

Ingredients:

For the Salad:

- 8 cups kale leaves, stems removed and chopped
- 1 cup blueberries
- 1/2 cup red onion, thinly sliced
- 1/2 cup feta cheese, crumbled
- 1/4 cup sunflower seeds

For the Lemon Poppyseed Dressing:

- 1/4 cup olive oil
- 2 tablespoons lemon juice
- 1 tablespoon honey
- 1 teaspoon Dijon mustard
- 1 teaspoon poppy seeds
- Salt and pepper to taste

Nutritional Information (per serving):

- **Carbs:** 25g
- **Sodium:** 120mg
- **Fats:** 15g
- **Protein:** 7g

Instructions:

1. Remove the stems from the kale leaves and chop them into bite-sized pieces.
2. In a small bowl, whisk together olive oil, lemon juice, honey, Dijon mustard, poppy seeds, salt, and pepper. Set aside.
3. In a large bowl, massage the chopped kale with a small amount of the prepared dressing. This helps to soften the kale.
4. Add blueberries, thinly sliced red onion, crumbled feta cheese, and sunflower seeds to the massaged kale.
5. Drizzle the remaining dressing over the salad ingredients.
6. Gently toss the salad until all ingredients are well coated with the dressing.
7. Use extra-virgin olive oil for its anti-inflammatory properties.
8. Incorporate honey for sweetness, which may have anti-inflammatory benefits.
9. Include Dijon mustard for its potential anti-inflammatory effects.
10. Limit added salt to reduce sodium content.

<u>Strawberry and Avocado Quinoa Bowl</u>

Prep Time: 15 minutes | **Cook Time:** 15 minutes | **Servings:** 4

Ingredients:

- 1 cup quinoa, rinsed
- 2 cups water
- 1 pound strawberries, hulled and sliced
- 2 avocados, diced
- 1/4 cup red onion, finely chopped
- 1/4 cup fresh basil leaves, chopped
- 1/4 cup feta cheese, crumbled
- 2 tablespoons balsamic glaze
- 2 tablespoons extra-virgin olive oil
- Salt and pepper to taste

Nutritional Information (per serving):

- **Carbs:** 40g
- **Sodium:** 80mg
- **Fats:** 15g
- **Protein:** 8g

Instructions:

1. In a medium saucepan, combine the quinoa and water. Bring to a boil, then reduce heat to low, cover, and simmer for 15 minutes or until the quinoa is cooked and water is absorbed.
2. Fluff the cooked quinoa with a fork and let it cool to room temperature.
3. Hull and slice the strawberries.
4. Dice the avocados.
5. Finely chop the red onion.
6. Chop the fresh basil leaves.
7. In a large bowl, combine the cooled quinoa, sliced strawberries, diced avocados, chopped red onion, chopped basil leaves, and crumbled feta cheese.
8. Drizzle the balsamic glaze and extra-virgin olive oil over the quinoa mixture.
9. Season the bowl with salt and pepper to taste. Gently toss to combine all the ingredients.
10. Use extra-virgin olive oil for its anti-inflammatory properties.
11. Include fresh basil for potential anti-inflammatory benefits.
12. Limit added salt to reduce sodium content.
13. Choose a balsamic glaze with reduced sodium or make your own to control salt intake.

Berry and Coconut Yogurt Parfait

Prep Time: 10 minutes | **Cook Time:** 0 minutes | **Servings:** 4

Ingredients:

- 2 cups plain Greek yogurt
- 1 cup mixed berries (blueberries, strawberries, raspberries)
- 1/2 cup shredded coconut
- 1/4 cup almond butter
- 2 tablespoons honey
- 1 teaspoon vanilla extract
- 1/4 cup granola (optional, for topping)

Nutritional Information (per serving):

- **Carbs:** 25g
- **Sodium:** 40mg
- **Fats:** 15g
- **Protein:** 12g

Instructions:

1. In a bowl, mix Greek yogurt, almond butter, honey, and vanilla extract until well combined.
2. In serving glasses or bowls, start with a layer of the yogurt mixture.
3. Top the yogurt with a layer of mixed berries and shredded coconut.
4. Repeat the layering process until the glasses are filled, finishing with a layer of berries and coconut on top.
5. If desired, sprinkle a small amount of granola on the top layer for added crunch.
6. Choose plain Greek yogurt for its probiotic and anti-inflammatory properties.
7. Opt for unsweetened shredded coconut to reduce added sugars.
8. Include berries for their high antioxidant content.
9. Use almond butter for its potential anti-inflammatory benefits.
10. Limit added honey to reduce sugar intake.
11. Prepare the parfait components separately and assemble just before serving to maintain the freshness of the layers.

Blackberry and Mint Infused Water

Prep Time: 5 minutes | **Cook Time:** 0 minutes | **Servings:** 4

Ingredients:

- 2 cups blackberries
- 1 bunch fresh mint leaves
- 1 lemon, sliced
- 1.5 liters water (filtered or still mineral water)

Nutritional Information (per serving):

- **Carbs:** 12g
- **Sodium:** 10mg
- **Fats:** 0g
- **Protein:** 1g

Instructions:

1. Wash the blackberries, mint leaves, and lemon thoroughly.
2. In a large pitcher, muddle the blackberries and mint leaves gently. This helps release their flavors.
3. Add the sliced lemon to the pitcher.
4. Pour the water into the pitcher over the muddled blackberries, mint, and lemon slices.
5. Stir the ingredients together using a long spoon. Place the pitcher in the refrigerator to chill for at least 2 hours or overnight.
6. Before serving, you can strain the infused water to remove the fruit and mint pieces or leave them in for a more intense flavor.
7. Choose still mineral water or filtered water without added sugars or artificial additives.
8. Include fresh mint for its potential anti-inflammatory properties.
9. Blackberries are rich in antioxidants, contributing to potential anti-inflammatory benefits.
10. Lemon adds a burst of Vitamin C and potential anti-inflammatory properties.
11. This infused water is naturally low in sodium.

Mixed Berry Sorbet with Mint

Prep Time: 10 minutes | **Cook Time:** 0 minutes | **Freeze Time:** 4 hours | **Servings:** 4

Ingredients:

- 3 cups mixed berries (strawberries, blueberries, raspberries)
- 1/4 cup fresh mint leaves
- 1/4 cup honey or maple syrup
- 1 tablespoon lemon juice

Nutritional Information (per serving):

- **Carbs:** 25g
- **Sodium:** 5mg
- **Fats:** 0g
- **Protein:** 1g

Instructions:

1. Wash and hull the strawberries. Ensure all berries are clean and free of stems.
2. In a blender, combine the mixed berries, fresh mint leaves, honey or maple syrup, and lemon juice.
3. Blend the ingredients until you achieve a smooth and well-combined mixture.
4. If a smoother texture is desired, you can strain the berry mixture to remove seeds. This step is optional.
5. Pour the blended mixture into a shallow pan or dish.
6. Place the pan in the freezer and let the sorbet freeze for about 4 hours or until firm.
7. Once frozen, use a fork to scrape the sorbet to create a granita-like texture.
8. Serve the mixed berry sorbet in bowls or glasses. Garnish with additional fresh mint leaves.
9. Choose honey or maple syrup for sweetness, both of which may have anti-inflammatory benefits.
10. Berries, especially strawberries and blueberries, are known for their high antioxidant and anti-inflammatory properties.
11. Mint leaves contribute potential anti-inflammatory benefits.

Berry and Almond Butter Smoothie

Prep Time: 5 minutes | **Cook Time:** 0 minutes | **Servings:** 2

Ingredients:

- 1 cup mixed berries (strawberries, blueberries, raspberries)
- 1 banana, peeled
- 2 tablespoons almond butter
- 1 cup almond milk (unsweetened)
- 1 tablespoon chia seeds
- Ice cubes (optional)

Nutritional Information (per serving):

- **Carbs:** 30g
- **Sodium:** 80mg
- **Fats:** 15g
- **Protein:** 5g

Instructions:

1. Wash the mixed berries and hull the strawberries. Peel the banana.
2. In a blender, combine the mixed berries, banana, almond butter, almond milk, and chia seeds.
3. Blend the ingredients until you achieve a smooth and creamy consistency.
4. If the smoothie is too thick, add more almond milk, or if it's too thin, add ice cubes and blend again.
5. Choose unsweetened almond milk for its anti-inflammatory properties.
6. Berries, especially strawberries and blueberries, are rich in antioxidants and known for their potential anti-inflammatory benefits.
7. Almond butter provides healthy fats and may have anti-inflammatory effects.
8. Prepare individual smoothie packs by portioning out the berries, banana, almond butter, and chia seeds into freezer-safe bags. Store them in the freezer, and when ready to make a smoothie, just blend with almond milk.

Grilled Turkey Burgers with Berry Compote

Prep Time: 15 minutes | **Cook Time:** 15 minutes | **Servings:** 4

Ingredients:

For the Turkey Burgers:

- 1 pound lean ground turkey
- 1/4 cup finely chopped red onion
- 1 clove garlic, minced
- 1 teaspoon dried oregano
- Salt and pepper to taste
- Whole-grain burger buns

For the Berry Compote:

- 1 cup mixed berries (strawberries, blueberries, raspberries)
- 1 tablespoon balsamic vinegar
- 1 tablespoon honey
- Fresh mint leaves for garnish

Nutritional Information (per serving):

- **Carbs:** 30g
- **Sodium:** 250mg
- **Fats:** 10g
- **Protein:** 25g

Instructions:

1. Preheat the grill to medium-high heat.
2. In a bowl, combine the ground turkey, finely chopped red onion, minced garlic, dried oregano, salt, and pepper. Mix until well combined.
3. Divide the turkey mixture into 4 equal portions and shape them into burger patties.
4. Grill the turkey burgers for about 6-8 minutes per side or until they reach an internal temperature of 165°F (74°C).
5. In a small saucepan, combine the mixed berries, balsamic vinegar, and honey. Cook over medium heat until the berries break down and the mixture thickens, stirring occasionally.
6. Choose lean ground turkey for a heart-healthy option.
7. Include garlic for its potential anti-inflammatory effects.
8. Opt for whole-grain burger buns for added fiber and anti-inflammatory benefits.
9. Use honey for sweetness, which may have anti-inflammatory benefits.
10. Limit added salt in both the turkey burgers and compote to reduce sodium content.
11. Place the grilled turkey burgers on whole-grain buns and top them with the berry compote. Garnish with fresh mint leaves.

Berry and Walnut Stuffed Acorn Squash

Prep Time: 15 minutes | **Cook Time:** 45 minutes | **Servings:** 4

Ingredients:

- 2 acorn squash, halved and seeds removed
- 1 cup mixed berries (blueberries, raspberries, blackberries)
- 1/2 cup walnuts, chopped
- 1/4 cup dried cranberries
- 1/4 cup fresh parsley, chopped
- 2 tablespoons olive oil
- 1 tablespoon balsamic vinegar
- 1 teaspoon maple syrup
- Salt and pepper to taste

Nutritional Information (per serving):

- **Carbs:** 40g
- **Sodium:** 15mg
- **Fats:** 15g
- **Protein:** 5g

Instructions:

1. Preheat the oven to 375°F (190°C).
2. Cut the acorn squash in half, scoop out the seeds, and brush the cut sides with olive oil. Place them cut side down on a baking sheet.
3. Roast the acorn squash in the preheated oven for about 40-45 minutes or until the squash is fork-tender.
4. In a bowl, combine mixed berries, chopped walnuts, dried cranberries, fresh parsley, olive oil, balsamic vinegar, maple syrup, salt, and pepper.
5. Choose olive oil for its anti-inflammatory properties.
6. Berries, especially blueberries and blackberries, are rich in antioxidants and known for their potential anti-inflammatory benefits.
7. Walnuts provide omega-3 fatty acids with potential anti-inflammatory effects.
8. Dried cranberries add sweetness with potential anti-inflammatory benefits.
9. Once the acorn squash halves are cooked, flip them over and fill each cavity with the berry and walnut mixture.
10. Place the stuffed acorn squash back in the oven for an additional 5-7 minutes to heat the filling.
11. Garnish with additional fresh parsley if desired and serve immediately.
12. Prepare the filling in advance and store it separately. When ready to serve, reheat the filling and stuff it into freshly roasted acorn squash halves.

Mixed Berry and Quinoa Breakfast Casserole

Prep Time: 15 minutes | **Cook Time:** 45 minutes | **Servings:** 6

Ingredients:

- 1 cup quinoa, rinsed
- 2 cups almond milk (unsweetened)
- 4 large eggs
- 1/4 cup maple syrup
- 1 teaspoon vanilla extract
- 1 teaspoon ground cinnamon
- 1/2 teaspoon baking powder
- 2 cups mixed berries (blueberries, strawberries, raspberries)
- 1/4 cup sliced almonds
- Fresh mint leaves for garnish (optional)

Nutritional Information (per serving):

- **Carbs:** 40g
- **Sodium:** 100mg
- **Fats:** 15g
- **Protein:** 10g

Instructions:

1. Preheat the oven to 375°F (190°C). Grease a baking dish with cooking spray.
2. In a saucepan, combine quinoa and almond milk. Bring to a boil, then reduce heat to low, cover, and simmer for 15 minutes or until quinoa is cooked.
3. In a large bowl, whisk together eggs, maple syrup, vanilla extract, ground cinnamon, and baking powder.
4. Add the cooked quinoa to the egg mixture and mix well.

Chapter 10: Sustainably Embracing the Anti-Inflammatory Lifestyle

Critical Tips for Long-Term Success

Adopting an anti-inflammatory lifestyle is a transformative journey that demands dedication and flexibility. Here are some essential tips to guarantee long-term success:

1. Educate Yourself: Gain a thorough understanding of the science behind inflammation and the benefits of an anti-inflammatory diet. This knowledge can serve as a strong motivator to help you stay committed to the diet. Stay informed by reading books, attending workshops, and following credible sources.

2. Start Slowly: Gradually incorporate anti-inflammatory foods into your diet rather than making sudden and drastic adjustments. This approach ensures a smooth and lasting transition.

3. Diversify Your Diet: Incorporating a diverse range of foods into your meals helps ensure you receive a balanced set of nutrients and adds some excitement to your dining experience. Try out various recipes, ingredients, and cooking methods to keep things interesting.

4. Plan and Prepare: To stay on track, plan and prepare your meals in advance. Allocate time every week to plan your meals, create shopping lists, and prepare your ingredients. Having nutritious meals prepared in advance helps resist the urge to choose less healthy alternatives.

5. Listen to Your Body: Be mindful of your body's reactions to various foods. Everyone is unique, and what may be effective for one person may not yield the same results for someone else. Modify your diet to suit your individual needs and preferences.

6. Stay Hydrated: Drink plenty of water to reduce inflammation and support overall health. Strive to consume at least eight glasses of water daily and consider the potential anti-inflammatory advantages of herbal teas.

Building Healthy Habits

Establishing healthy habits is the cornerstone of sustaining an anti-inflammatory lifestyle. Here's a step-by-step guide to developing and maintaining these habits:

1. Set Attainable Goals: Set realistic and measurable goals to maintain your motivation. Begin by making minor modifications, like adding one anti-inflammatory meal daily, and then gradually build on them.

2. Establish a Routine: Consistency plays a vital role in developing new habits. Create a consistent schedule that incorporates meal preparation, physical activity, and self-care practices. Maintaining a consistent routine is crucial, but it's also important to be flexible when necessary.

3. Find Enjoyable Activities: Participate in physical activities that bring you happiness, such as yoga, walking, swimming, or dancing. Regular exercise is beneficial for reducing inflammation and promoting overall well-being.

4. Engage Your Family and Friends: Keep your loved ones informed about your journey. Invite them to join you in adopting an anti-inflammatory lifestyle. Cooking and eating together can be a fun and supportive way to stay on track.

5. Prioritize Self-Care: Stress can potentially worsen inflammation, so it's crucial to include self-care activities in your daily routine. Engaging in activities such as meditation, deep breathing exercises, and spending time in nature can be beneficial for managing stress levels.

6. Track Your Progress: Keep a journal to record your meals, physical activity, mood, and any health changes. Tracking your progress can help you recognize patterns, acknowledge achievements, and make any needed modifications.

7. Stay Positive: Maintain a positive mindset and concentrate on your progress instead of dwelling on your sacrifices. Acknowledge and appreciate the small victories in your journey towards an anti-inflammatory lifestyle. Remember to reflect on the positive benefits you are experiencing along the way.

Conclusion

Committing to an anti-inflammatory lifestyle is a way to prioritize your long-term health and well-being. Throughout this cookbook, we have delved into the fundamentals of anti-inflammatory eating, offered practical meal prep techniques, and provided various mouthwatering recipes to decrease inflammation while promoting overall well-being.

By incorporating these principles into your daily routine, you are actively working towards reducing chronic inflammation, effectively managing stress, and enhancing your overall quality of life. Remember that maintaining this lifestyle requires careful planning, preparation, and consistent effort. Take advantage of the knowledge and tools provided in this cookbook to develop a well-rounded, diverse, and pleasurable approach that aligns with your health objectives.

Take a moment to acknowledge your progress and the positive changes you've experienced. Continue to discover new culinary delights, try out different recipes, and stay up-to-date with the latest findings in anti-inflammatory nutrition. Above all, pay close attention to your body and adjust your approach accordingly.

We appreciate your decision to select "The Complete Anti-Inflammatory Meal Prep Cookbook" as your trusted companion. We hope it motivates you to keep moving forward with a sense of assurance and excitement, nurturing a more vibrant and content version of yourself. Here's to a life filled with vibrant health and delicious, nourishing meals!

Recipes Index

Turmeric-Ginger Lentil Soup 82

Turmeric-Lemon Grilled Chicken Thighs 90

Turmeric-Lime Coconut Energy Bites 99

Turmeric-Spiced Quinoa Patties 88

Turmeric-Spiced Sweet Potato Soup 96

W

Walnut and Cranberry Stuffed Acorn Squash 75

Walnut-Crusted Chicken Salad with Raspberry Vinaigrette 68

Walnut-Crusted Chicken Tenders with Zucchini Noodles 40

Z

Zucchini and Spinach Egg Muffins 50